PARKINSON'S

A LOVE STORY
WITH DEMENTIA
FOR DESSERT

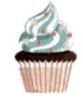

AVA S. BUTLER

Parkinson's: A Love Story with Dementia for Dessert

Copyright © 2019 Ava S. Butler. All rights reserved. No part of this book may be reproduced or retransmitted in any form or by any means without the written permission of the publisher.

Published by Wheatmark®
2030 East Speedway Boulevard, Suite 106
Tucson, Arizona 85719 USA
www.wheatmark.com

ISBN: 978-1-62787-644-5 (paperback)
ISBN: 978-1-62787-645-2 (ebook)
LCCN: 2018909531

This book is dedicated to my dear husband and soulmate, Richard Ping,

and to all his caregivers and our many friends and family who love and support us through every step of our journey.

We are blessed to have you all in our lives.

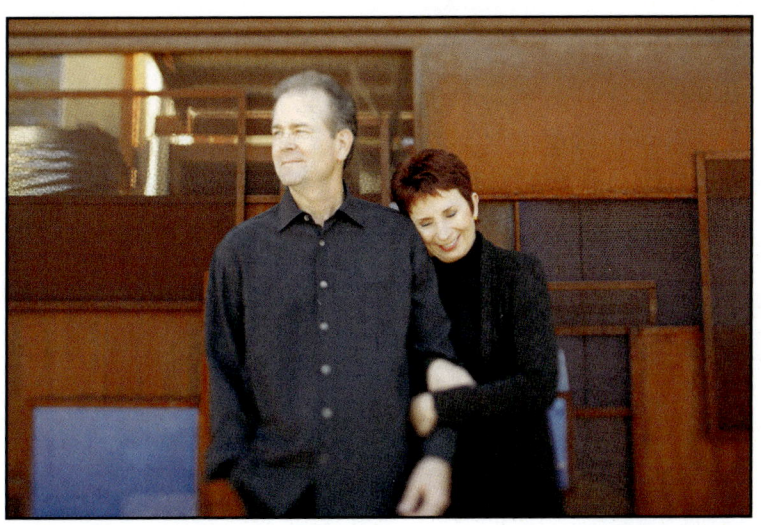

PHOTO BY PURPLE NICKEL

Meet the True Bad Boys

Parkinson's disease is a degenerative neurological disorder that affects one in one hundred people over age sixty. Men have a somewhat higher risk than women. While the average age at onset is around sixty, some people are diagnosed at forty or younger.

Parkinson's is a disorder of the central nervous system that results from the loss of cells in the brain that make dopamine. Dopamine is responsible for transmitting signals that allow for coordination of movement. Loss of dopamine leaves patients less able to direct or control their movement.

People with Parkinson's disease can also experience difficulties outside of movement, including memory problems and in later stages, even dementia (significant memory/thinking changes that impact daily life). And while Parkinson's itself can be the cause of dementia, there's a lesser-known but related cause of dementia called Lewy body dementia (LBD).

LBD is not as well-known as Alzheimer's, but it is the second most common form of dementia. Persistent and recurring visual hallucinations (seeing things that aren't there) are often an early symptom. More than 1.4 million Americans are impacted by LBD, but little public attention is paid to this lesser-known disorder.

The disease did get a boost in publicity when Robin Williams was diagnosed with LBD after his suicide in 2014, but far more public information is needed.

My dear husband, Richard, had both. At least this is what we know without an autopsy, which was the furthest thing from my mind at the moment when such a decision should have been made.

I learned all I know so far from the Michael J. Fox Foundation, the Lewy Body Dementia Association, much research, and Richard's doctors.

Here's the headline: These are horrible diseases that you wouldn't wish on your worst enemy. They are unwelcome invaders into your once normal and happy existence. They will wage a war that you will not win. Not yet, anyway. But there are tools to fight the battle.

I wrote this book as part of my own healing process. My goal is to help others on their journey with Parkinson's and LBD and to share the idea that love stories come in many forms.

The book is a combination of my journal, blogs, and reflections. It's not exactly a comedy, but I hope it will warm your heart.

More on bad boys later.

Meet Richard Ping

6 July 1991

On our wedding day, these were my vows to Richard:

Dearest Richard
I often wondered if it was true what they said
That my expectations were unrealistic and bold
But I knew it was better to live life alone than
  to compromise a dream
And when I met you, I knew why I had waited
I love who you are and what we've already
  become
And know our bond will only grow stronger
I'm graced by your love and will cherish you
  always
Grow old with me, Richard
The best is yet to come
Forever, Ava Sue

Our love did grow stronger. But we didn't really get a chance to grow old together.

Richard died when he was sixty-five.

He was diagnosed with Parkinson's on May 26,

2010, and he left the earth on March 26, 2017. Seven short and very long years.

We met in a bar through mutual friends on February 8, 1991. We spent that Friday night and the weekend together, and he moved in on Monday. We were married five months later. I was thirty-three, and Richard was thirty-nine. We met in Seattle and then moved to northern Italy, then London, San Diego, Tucson, Vancouver, and then back to Tucson.

I always thought we'd be the cute old couple walking hand in hand, still in love after all those years. Just like we were in this photograph, taken of us on Halloween 1992. Dying in our sleep at the exact same moment, our bodies entwined in a final embrace. But that's not the way it turned out.

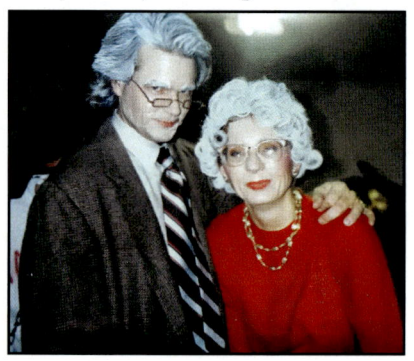

I'm grateful for the travels we had when we were young. "Travel when your legs work," we used to say. Now I say, "Travel when your legs and brain work."

Richard charmed people wherever we went with his handsome looks, easygoing attitude, and interest in other people and their lives. I called him the king of open-ended questions. He would find out things about people that others who had known them for years didn't know. When asked about his uncanny ability, he would simply say, "I asked questions and listened to the answers."

But we didn't expect the same openness from him. He was not one to share his feelings, hopes, fears, or disappointments. "He was not an open book, always unconventional, and a bit of a mystery. He was a kind person, gentle even, considerate and respectful." Those are his friend Steve's words. Richard had a fabulous sense of humor and drew people to him like a magnet.

Richard had been a star since the day he was born, a gifted athlete with a sharp mind. He was born to Marilyn and Vernon Ping on July 23, 1951, with one older brother, Jim. He was Dickie as a child, Dick when I met him, Riccardo when we lived in Italy, and Richard when we moved to London.

Meet nine-year-old Dickie, with his cousin Kathy and brother Jimmie. "Hey, Dickie, I like your bat." That would have been a good pickup line.

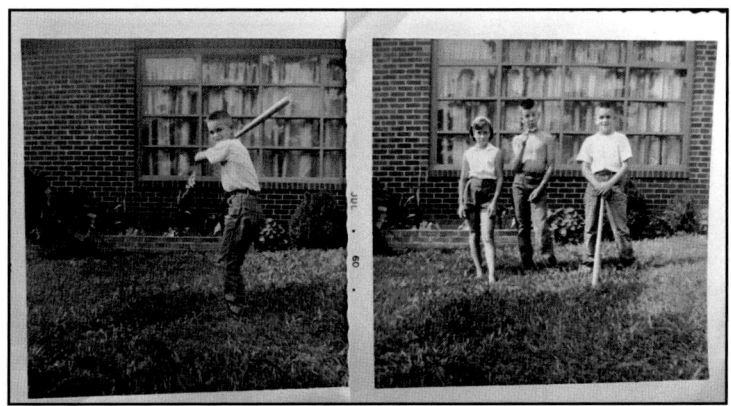

He was a gifted poet and writer. His first childhood

poem was about farts. He recited it often. It was clever and pretty amusing. I wish I'd had the sense to write it down.

Here's the poem he wrote for our wedding.

Wedding Dance

A whispered promise
Slows our step
Near motionless.
And knowing silence
Bends into our spin
Revolving web
And loving focus
To this wedding dance
We share.

RVP 7-6-91

We were soulmates. And still are, of course. But I won't get into that yet.

The Beginning of the End

22 March 2012

My husband has Parkinson's disease. When our neurologist, Dr. Sullivan, first said so back in May of 2010, my first thought was, *Damn, he was right.* Richard is a bit of a hypochondriac and has a tendency to exaggerate. He's thought he had bone cancer, skin cancer, and on and on, and when he said he had Parkinson's, I didn't believe him. But there was definitely something wrong, and our friends who didn't see him much noticed it more than I did.

Even back in 2009 and 2010 he was already starting to have trouble with his golf swing. His hand would shake slightly when he placed his ball on the tee and when he was holding his fork at the dinner table. He said he felt little twitches in his arm. He started acting out his dreams, which I just learned is due to a REM sleep behavior disorder; one of the strongest prediagnostic symptoms of Parkinson's, along with a lost sense of smell and subtle changes in cognition.

He saw phantasms by his bed at night. He would lose his train of thought, losing words and finding himself unable to complete sentences. I'd find things in strange places, like his cell phone in the cupboard. He had panic attacks that sent us to the emergency room for hours and hours.

In 2011, he got so paranoid that someone was plotting to get him as part of a sting operation that he would arrive at the airport to pick me up hours before my flight was to arrive. He was afraid to stay in the house by himself. If the doorbell rang, he would hide. "It's just a kid asking for money for his baseball team," I said. This was of no consolation. I thought he was developing a mental illness.

Now he's less productive by the day. No ambition. No gusto. Meanwhile, I continue to work my ass off. Not a good balance.

It might sound like I don't love him. But I do. More than anything. More every day.

18 April 2012

Today is a scary day. Richard wanted to transfer some money from one bank account to another. He should have transferred money from our personal savings to our personal checking. Instead, he transferred money to my business checking. "No problem," I said. "Just transfer the money from the business checking account back to personal checking." But there was a problem. Richard couldn't follow the logic. His mind got frozen. He needed help. But he couldn't understand it even with repeated explanations. And he was frustrated. "I used to be good at math."

And now I'm scared. Scared that he won't be able

to keep up. Scared that I will lose him and that he will lose his mind. And how will I pay for his care? How much will it take? Can I do it?

1 September 2012

It's all gone downhill a lot since then. He never transfers money. Won't ever again. It's sobering, really. He's very depressed today and has been a lot lately. He started working with Susan, his cognitive therapist, a few months ago, and the brain apps she recommended seem to help, but not enough. He does work on them for hours every day though. That's to his credit. His writing is eloquent when he writes. But he's not writing nearly often enough. He's trying, but I don't think he's trying his hardest. His body hurts all the time, mainly from the peripheral neuropathy, I think. I massage his feet and legs almost every day.

Maybe he is trying his hardest, but it might be the first time ever, except for basketball and golf. "Dickie, why don't you try?" That's what his grade school teacher said. Richard is one of those annoying people who is good at everything. He didn't have to try hard, and he's still better than almost anyone. This will be the time when he is going to have to try hard, and he still won't win. These are formidable invaders. I remind him that he has to try his hardest this time, but it's not helpful.

I really don't have anyone to talk to about this. Maybe I should find someone. I think of myself as a strong person, but I'm not sure how strong I can be or for how long. It's going to be a lifelong commitment. I love him so much. But it's different now.

I don't think I'm going to be able to travel for my work for very long. I've been a road warrior organizational development consultant for years. It's what I know and what I'm good at. So how can I make a lot of money without traveling? I must get serious about writing and finding another way. I wrote a book on meeting management skills back in 1995, and it did well. I can update and republish that as a start.

I think I should keep a better journal of what happens. I'm surprised to read that it was only April when the confusion over the bank accounts happened. It seems like a long, long time ago.

We're in London now for my work and have been since the end of May. It's good, but it would be better if Richard were home and getting more help, especially from Susan. Her help with memory and communication seems essential. It's the biggest challenge. Please don't take his brain, or mine either. If I were home, I'd smoke a big hit of pot. It's hard to cope.

24 December 2012

So much has changed this year. Richard's memory is a real challenge for him. He can't remember the date or year very accurately, even though we repeat it several times a day. The apps and writing exercises that Susan gives him are essential. They're good for me too. We've learned a lot about the brain; that's one benefit.

I worry about money more now. I know I can't keep traveling for too many more years, and I have to find a different way to make money. I really must start working on my book. I've been talking about it for almost a decade. I used to be much more laid-back about finding work. But I'm worried that we'll need to have a lot more money if Richard needs more care. Parkinson's is very expensive, even now. I don't know what we would do without health insurance and money for everything it doesn't cover. I'm grateful we can pay.

We're at the age when our friends are dying already. Shawn's husband, Doug, dropped dead of a heart attack. She's heartbroken. Our friend Sal tells us he has some rare form of bone marrow disease. This is sobering.

I don't feel angry with Richard anymore. I used to be frustrated about his lack of productivity. He is a great writer and was doing well writing stage plays after he sold his real estate appraisal business. But then he stopped. I thought it was because we moved back to the United States from London, where the theatre scene is awesome and where he was becoming well connected. But now I understand better. His diseases were in their early phases, but we didn't know.

There are times I see Richard sitting on the couch with a serious look on his face. When I ask what he is doing, he says, "I'm trying to figure out what is going on, but I can't." He knows his brain is changing. This is heartbreaking.

I cherish our time together. We don't know how long we'll have. He doesn't feel good often, and his communication is frequently unclear. I can usually decipher what he is talking about, but others can't all the time. But it's important to get out and try. He started taking the Exelon Patch for memory, and we'll see if that helps. Our neurologist tells us things will only get worse. This is very sobering.

Modern Medicine Failed Us and without Emotional Intelligence

April 2013

Richard and I were looking for so many ways to fight the inevitable—anything we could find to help him with his Parkinson's and dementia. We went to the University of Arizona's neurology department for insights.

It's a teaching hospital, so there were medical students there. They gave him the Montreal Cognitive Assessment, and he did shitty. Of course he did shitty—he has f'ing Parkinson's and dementia, and he wanted to stop. But the students didn't care. They had a test to perform, come hell or high water. They were unempathetic and not even conscious of the pain and humiliation taking that test was causing Richard. I cry as I write these words. For example, they asked him to repeat ten words. He couldn't remember ten words. He couldn't remember three, but they insisted on ten. It was demoralizing.

Later, when we talked to the doctor, he had nothing to offer us. I asked for leading-edge techniques such as hyperbaric oxygen and stem cell replacement therapy. He told us, without empathy, that there was no evidence that these things would make a long-term difference. He gave us nothing.

I was angry, Richard was defeated, and when we got into the car, we both cried hard. It was the only time I remember seeing Richard cry about his condition and ultimate fate. I still cry often, but he kept it inside after that.

Modern medicine failed us—and without emotional intelligence.

Even though I asked repeatedly, the neurologist's office never sent me a copy of the test results; if they had, I would share them with you now. But I'll show you an online example of what's on the test.

IMAGE: MARK P. MATTSON / FRONTIERS IN NEUROSCIENCE

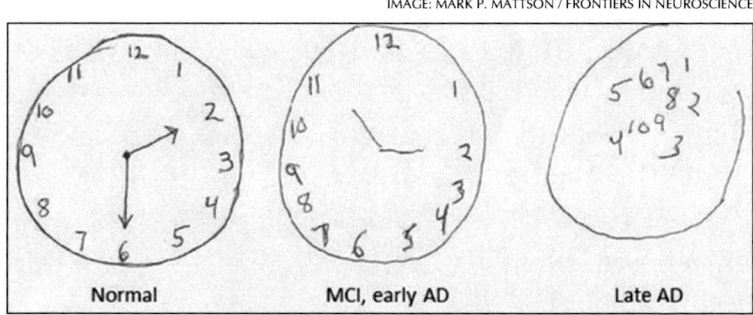

MCI=Mild Cognitive Impairment AD=Alzhiemer's Disease

Headline: It's hard to draw clocks when you have dementia.

Progress in the Wrong Direction

20 March 2013

It's the first day of spring already. Richard has been having a bad week, feeling poorly, and having difficulty accomplishing tasks. I really need to write in my journal more. This could be a good record of his situation. We're going to Dr. Ramsey, a naturopath in Scottsdale next week, and I pray that will help. We got our medical records from Dr. Sullivan in preparation, and the first page includes my comment: "I want my husband back." Well, he's not coming back. That makes me cry and feel very sad. I love him so much, and that won't change, but our lives have been changed forever.

I'm working to finish my book, and I have to be very serious about other ways to make money that don't take me away from home for long. Richard is totally dependent on others to make appointments for him and pay his bills.

I was afraid for him to drive himself to his golf lesson today. Sometimes he gets lost and goes the wrong way. Golf is so important to Richard, and he's really good at it. I'm not sure how much longer that will be true, though. Giving up golf will make him sad. Another loss in a long series of losses.

His communication is very obtuse. It's a guessing game to understand the content and purpose of what he says. No one told us that the dementia would happen, and no one seems to be able or willing to tell us what to expect. Or maybe I'm just not able to listen.

24 March 2013

Richard's new drug, Exelon, made him so sick today. He was very wobbly and shaky, with an upset stomach so bad he vomited. We had tickets to Festival en el Barrio today, but that is not going to happen. I really like that outdoor festival, and this is the last year that we could walk from our house. I feel sad that we can't go—particularly as I think this is going to happen to us more and more and more and more.

He's going to stop the Exelon, which is crap for Richard and the only pharmaceutical choice for saving his brain. This disease sucks.

16 April 2013

We spent the week last week at Dr. Ramsey's clinic, the Center for Natural Healing, with four days of hyperbaric oxygen therapy (HBOT) and glutathione intravenous treatments. I was very hopeful—praying—for a miraculous recovery, and Richard's peripheral neuropathy did get better. His communication was better, and his energy was higher. But not long after we left, his communication skills declined to their previous level. Yesterday, he drove himself to the massage therapist, to a building where he had been many times before and got lost both on the way there and on the way home. This is scary. I have to say that my hopes are lower, and I know that this is a long-term game. I need to be all that I can be and find a new way of making money. I need to have the best energy and as disciplined a focus as possible to support our efforts.

We got a new book that Dr. Ramsey uses called *You Can Heal Yourself*. I'm going to read it and learn everything I can. Maybe I'm part of the problem.

16 April 2014

Coincidentally, it's been a year to the day since I wrote anything here. And today is a very difficult day. It's the day I realized that one day I could be part of an assisted suicide. There will be a point in the future, maybe not so far away, when Richard won't be able to take it anymore.

I worry all the time about being able to make enough money and having enough time to work. Assisting Richard is now almost a full-time job.

But let's recap what happened over the last year.

We moved last May to a condo that is 'lock and leave' and much less expensive than anywhere else we've ever lived. But it has good bones and a good view, and we like it here. Our house on S. Ninth Avenue had an open floor plan, but this has lots of rooms and a long hallway. Bad idea. Richard gets lost in our new house every day. We're planning to blast out the kitchen wall and make an open floor plan in the front of the house. That will help in the front of the house, but it won't help with the hallway and the too-many doors.

I started work on my book *Mission Critical Meetings: 81 Practical Facilitation Techniques* over a year ago, and it's now in the final phases before being published. I'm blogging the techniques. These are small steps to making a living without being on the road.

I took a consulting job in Oklahoma City last July, and Richard insisted that he could stay home alone. It went well for one day. Then he started having terrible hallucinations. Not the nice 1960s kind, either. He got spooked and went outside, where he thought it was safer. Mind you, it's really hot in Tucson in July. Our kind neighbors, Allen and Teresa, rescued him and brought him inside. He was too scared of the "bad boys" in the house, but they assured him they were gone. They prepared a frozen pizza for him, which he immediately dropped upside down on the carpet. They made him another one and got him to drink more water. Thankfully I was flying home that night. When I got home, he was on the lookout from the back terrace. I was so grateful he was there and not running away from the bad boys again. God, that sucked. I wasn't happy about pizza all over the carpet, but that was the least of my worries.

The next week, Richard's brother, Jim, came to the rescue, jumping on a plane from Vancouver so I could keep working. I am so grateful. I got a message from my next-door neighbor when I got off the plane in Dallas saying that Richard was out on the front terrace, yelling at people who weren't there. It was still early, and I called to wake Jim up; he immediately went outside, but Richard was inconsolable. It wasn't until Jim started to cry that Richard was able to change his perspective to focus on Jim instead of the imaginary enemies. This is really hard for Jim too—seeing his little brother with so much stress and fear.

After Jim left, I got our painter, Paul, to stay with him during the day, but Richard was on his own at night. Disaster. One night he was frightened by bad boys in the house again and drove the car to a hotel that was really a dorm. These bad boys were especially big and tough and had tattoos on their teeth. The UA campus police got involved, and luckily I was able to reach Paul who came to get him, or else he would have spent the night in a hospital or jail.

Richard doesn't drive anymore, and I was impressed that he could even start our new car on his own. It's a Prius. Our Lexus was totaled in a car accident. Not our fault, but another trauma.

LSVT Big and Loud (excellent exercise programs for Parkinson's), lymphatic massages, glutathione drips, and another therapist, Christina Romano, are new additions. Christina has been an enormous help. She has helped him manage his fears in general and his hallucinations in particular.

I'm looking for strength. Our meditations are very

helpful. My favorite centering thoughts: I am open to the presence of miracles. I choose abundance.

I feel that we should take our safari for my sixtieth birthday in 2017, before I'm sixty. Just in case.

21 June 2014

What a crazy two months. Richard's condition took a turn for the worse. He was really out of it when our friend Andrea came for the weekend of May 10. The next week, he was incontinent (a delightful Parkinson's side effect) and peed in the bed twice in his sleep, once standing up to pee on the bed, and another time he peed on a bunch of clean clothes that he pulled off the drying rack. He then had to wear Depends 24/7 and needed complete help showering and getting onto and off the toilet. I have to wipe him. He shit on the floor once and in the shower twice and had terrible diarrhea in his Depends once because he couldn't find the bathroom in time. He went to the utility room instead and got stuck. F'ing long hallway with five doors. That's four doors too many. Now, constipation has become a real problem and is starting to take over our lives. (You guessed it, yet another one of Parkinson's many gifts.)

We had to cancel appointments with friends at the last minute several times starting in mid-May. He also refused to get into the HBOT chamber or have a massage with Shannon, even though we were already in her massage room.

On May 25, he got spooked in the parking lot of

the Safeway and refused to get in the car with me. He called for help to real and imaginary people and ran away from me with a cart. A kind man came to my rescue near the gas station, and I had to call the police because Richard was completely unmanageable. The police drove him home, as Richard refused to get in the car with me, and then he chose to go to the emergency room instead of staying home. He ended up staying in the hospital for two nights for surveillance and also having a twenty-four-hour-long EEG.

He took Seroquel for awhile; that diminished paranoid delusions, and his hallucinations were much more controlled, but his Parkinsonian symptoms increased so we had to stop. Rats.

He talks of death and suicide constantly and requires nonstop supervision. We hired a caregiver, Liz, to help me, and she started on May 28. She's been a huge help.

What Richard Sees: Insight into the Hallucinations Associated with Lewy Body Dementia

Persistent and recurring visual hallucinations are often an early symptom of LBD. This was true for Richard. Not all LBD hallucinations are fear based, but Richard's were. His ability to communicate clearly has been impacted, and sometimes words come out in an unusual and surprisingly poetic way.

Between 2013 and 2014, I documented, as clearly as I could, exactly what Richard told me he saw. I share what he told me as a way of providing insights to those whose lives are impacted by this devastating disease.

At the time, we knew he had Parkinson's, but we knew nothing about LBD. The hallucinations and dementia were far more difficult to manage than his physical symptoms. Now that his disease has progressed, his hallucinations have become more manageable and less frequent. But LBD remains our biggest challenge.

When Richard is having hallucinations, I try to do the following:

- Respect what he sees. Dismissing his reality is

not helpful and can actually make it appear that I am not trustworthy.

- Remind him that we are safe and secure and that everyone is on our side.
- Ask him to look in my eyes. This can help ground him. Remind him that I love him and we are safe and secure.
    - If I'm part of the hallucination, however, and am perceived to be involved in some conspiracy, I need to back off and give him some space.
- Ask him to describe what he sees. Sometimes this causes him to focus a bit more. What he sees can give me insights into how he is feeling. Anxiety produces scary hallucinations, but if he is calm and secure, the hallucinations tend to be positive.
- Improvise to turn the negative situation into one with a positive outcome. For example, "It first looked like it was a bad guy, but he's actually very friendly and on our side," or "I saw that guy before, and he's harmless and is actually here to help keep us safe."
- Tell him that he can instruct the people to back off and leave him alone.
- Walk slowly toward the hallucination and tell the 'people' Richard is seeing that it's time for them to go away now.

- Move and talk slowly and calmly. Fast movements cause higher anxiety.
- Be mindful of my own emotions. My own frustration, anger, or anxiety will make things worse.

Here's what Richard experienced as written from his own words:

There are people who come into our house uninvited, and they are not always friendly.

There are so many bad boys, and they are both black and white; some have tattoos. These people might hurt us and others. Richard is in range of them. If Richard tells them to go away, they may hurt generations of people.

Sometimes there are a lot of people on the balconies. Whole families and generations live outside, where the garages are. They sleep during the day. They could be political refugees and protected by the government.

Once one of them, a punk, tried to get in the house, and Richard had to physically push him out. He pushed back; then Richard pushed back again harder, and he went away.

· · · · ·

The plants on the balcony can turn into short people.

Sometimes a family of dwarfs stays in our house. A girl wearing all leather, including a leather mask, accompanies them. Everything about her is hard. One day she was standing by our bed, looking Richard over. She stayed a long time before leaving.

· · · · ·

Our totem pole is particularly interesting, as frequently people live inside. It is hard to tell if the real totem is on the floor or in the nearby mirror.

Recently Richard saw an old man and a woman walking into the totem. They were thirty-seven feet tall and twelve inches short. They went inside to sleep for free. The old man didn't want to do it. It's irresponsible. But the woman said he had to.

There is a woman who has had her lips cut off by someone mean. This is very disturbing. She sometimes lives in the totem and lingers in the house and on the balcony. Richard feels sorry for her.

There was a young woman who came in the house a lot a few months ago. She had a crush on Richard. She hasn't been around much lately.

· · · · ·

There is a war being fought outside the walls of our condo complex in the direction of Sixth Street and also behind the garages. There are pieces of military machinery and people outside.

There are commandos who practice war in the

trees. Their techniques are advanced, and they use technology. The quality of display after they work is phenomenal. They each have different systems.

There are up to twenty-four commandos total in the trees at any time. The time that they stay varies. They have fighting dogs who are killer strong and are also guide dogs.

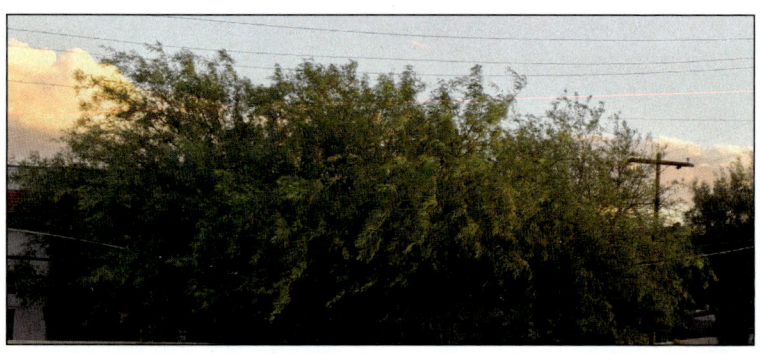

One guy in the group has binoculars. He is the general and is more powerful.

The commandos represent the future of America. They are young. They are a special band. Everyone who works here knows their lives are important.

They can stay for years and never be touched. If you look into their eyes, you can see that they are not unjust.

They are training for the end of the earth. We need to read a lot about history to know how to close the nuttles. They make the rich feel fear. Fear of invasion.

There is pressure against us and other groups. Anything could happen. We are in a danger period.

Why would the military not try to do something dangerous?

There are two tribes on the right-hand side—hundreds with warfare available. It could all be parked outside. It's a great place to live. Everyone trusts.

How many places like this have the ability to strike and find people to blow up?

Many people don't buy it. There are always people who can break the dam. It's hard to think about it.

This is all fake information. But what if it isn't?

The most overwhelming thing for Richard is this: "Where are these people coming from? What have I gotten myself into? I don't want to give them a ticket to Freetown and end up in an institution."

He asks, "What are they about? Why us?"

· · · · ·

It's been rather quiet around here for the last few months. Occasional people come in the house at night, but they go away when we turn on the lights and look around for them.

But yesterday was a very busy day. It started with a man sleeping and eating in our bedroom. Richard woke me up to look at him. But when we turned on the lights, he was gone. He was very fast.

And then there were a group of them in the closet—a whole bunch of them crowded in. They worked for the military and were there to protect us from the technology. They're on our side. They stayed longer.

They never really leave, actually. They're around even when you can't see them. They can disappear into the walls, no problem.

· · · · ·

The plants on the south balcony turned into little children again. Today they are musicians, and they played for everyone down below. People danced to their music.

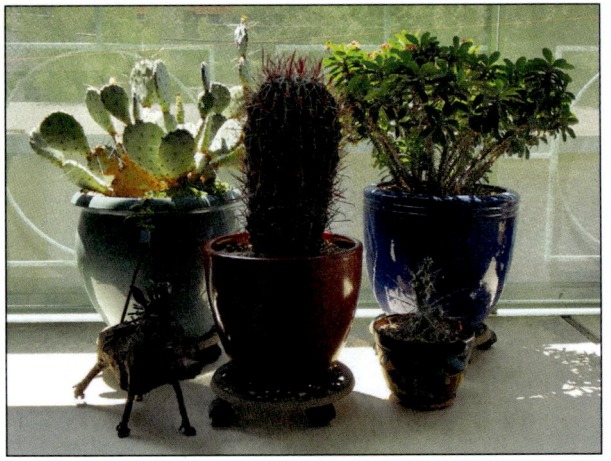

· · · · ·

Next, a woman appeared in the corner of the dining room. She was old enough to influence. She wore a red patterned dress, and her arms were hooks. Her real arms were gone. She left when I walked in the room. Richard tried to warn me to slow down so as not to scare her, but it was too late.

· · · · ·

There are a lot of conspiracies around. For example, most people would not expect that there is a prostitution ring right here in our condo complex, an over-fifty-five community. We don't talk about this often, as it is very dangerous. It's unwise to even write about it. It's unacceptable to say this.

· · · · ·

There is a rock band here to perform on our neighbor's patio. There are a lot of players—ten to fifteen. They look scruffy. It oils up the neighborhood. Their technician is unbelievably talented. Their equipment is weathered by the road. But the technician ensures there are no hitches, and its state of the art—as much as it can be. The setup is incredible, with a great stage and performance area.

· · · · ·

Our neighbors travel a lot and are out of town. African kings live there when they are gone. We shouldn't tell them; they would be jealous.

· · · · ·

Richard says he once had a massive hallucination and didn't quite have control. He lost some wheels along the road. He can't say more at this time.

· · · · ·

There are people in the trees preparing for a thank-you tour. They are a mature group. They're salacious people. No, change that to "Scooby-dooby-doo."

One guy is a huge size. The skinniest is also the smallest. He can't get off the lift. They all have brand-new shoes. It looks good for a getaway. They're moving out over the stage. It's a great before-and-after show. The people were born to be here.

The two orange trees on the left turned into a single giant horse. A part of the manicured shrubs turned into a pregnant woman—one without fornication because she couldn't dance. But she could …

Robadia. Rub it in. Robots. Tonight there could be robots.

· · · · ·

Richard says he had a couple of discoveries today. One of them involves butter. He couldn't say more.

There was a family inside our house today. There was a father and a mother and two to four children—little ones. They wore distinctive clothing. They stayed in the dining room area 75 percent of the time.

Richard had an aggressive moment with them, and it was a mistake. A full lease tire. A basic butter design. They were angry when he told them they had gone far enough. It's the fifth time they've been here.

"You're making this up," I say.

"No," says Richard, "that would be immature."

· · · · ·

Today Richard has forgotten my name. He thinks it's James Stephen Ping, his brother's name. Then he calls me Damaged Portilla. It sounds so sexy, he says. He forgot his name too. "My name? How would I ever know that?" he says, baffled by the thought of it.

· · · · ·

"I'm scared shitless," he says. "What will it take to go from scared shitless to safe and secure? Six more inches and the penitentiary. I'm going to get some trouble off this. You'll be able to hear me through transfer skills. It's a one-minute walk to find out."

•••••

Twelve motoring
Good bones in the body
Pay what you can
Carry a lot home
Super freight

•••••

Richard is using hyperbaric oxygen therapy (HBOT) to support his healing. It's a large oxygen tank that can seat up to six people. He stays inside for an hour at a time. On Monday he told me it was very crowded. In addition to him and the two other patients inside, a family of five pushed their way in uninvited.

And on Tuesday, in addition to Richard and the one other woman inside, there were two annoying flies and two airplanes. This made for a stressful hour.

•••••

Ava: Why are you so blue today?

Richard: I tried to get orange, but it wasn't available.

•••••

There are thirty people, and they're looking for magis pentifores. This is exciting. We stalk the house, looking for them. Here's the first one now. You've got to see this. There is a green one and a white one. They have no bearings or beepers. They can't hear us, but they can speak with each other. They speak English, but we can't hear them.

· · · · ·

Look at the green grass, on the ground where it is supposed to be. Freedom tatem toe. They've got a deer. The guy with the black shirt has it. It's probably in the back of the house.

We have to go get the Toetoa team. We don't know who they are exactly, so it could be difficult. Oops, no need now—they are here.

· · · · ·

Turn yourself over to a lord. I strongly suggest the turbo lite one.

· · · · ·

This is the easiest place in America to look for the girl right now. She's been victimized and has a child. She's standing right here in the kitchen. If she has powers, they are for our city.

· · · · ·

There is a man here again, a bad man. Dirt pack dolts. The people are under siege. My computer is an Etch A Sketch. Stop writing and look for the cylinder. Shut up; rub up. I want you to simmer and enjoy their jay.

· · · · ·

I am like a trading stamp.

· · · · ·

We've got to go; there is going to be a blast, and we're going to die. We could have died yesterday, but they passed the money through today. How tricky is that? About $4 million dollars goes to the winner. We don't know who won yet.

With car keys we can move from one place to another. Skip tumor; here we go. You got to take better care of your kids.

· · · · ·

Ava: Try to close your mouth. It's been gaping open lately.

Richard: Well, I've done a lot of walking.

· · · · ·

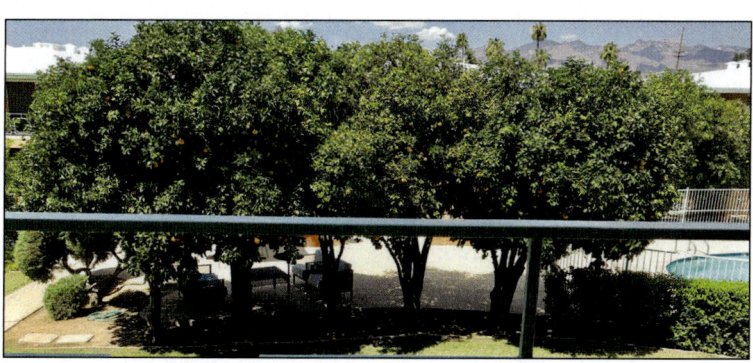

The common area outside our balcony often turns into a stage. There are stage plays there with a lot of people.

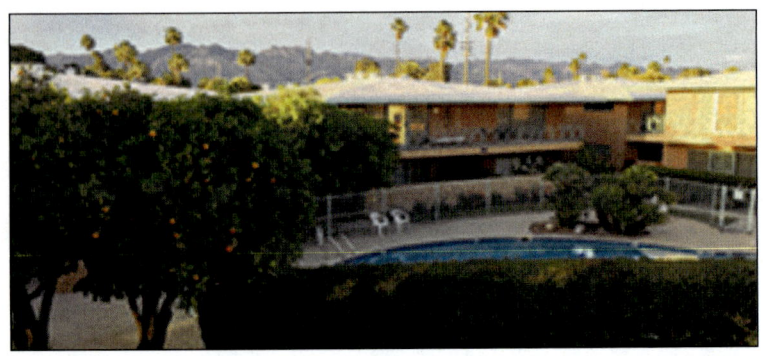

Sometimes there are weddings. The white chairs near the pool can turn into brides, and the shadows from the orange trees house lots of people. They seem to be moved by the sun and the wind. The rooftops are snow-covered mountains.

Richard usually likes the theatre and concerts outside. When he tells the people to go away, they come sneaking back. They like living here.

Peeing Our Way to Assisted Living

9 December 2014

Things are getting worse. Richard was incontinent at night again and can't understand that he needs to use the toilet not the floor. Damn you, Parkinson's and dementia. We've had several more accidents where he has peed the floor, including three times on our new carpeting.

Last night he fought me for twenty minutes to sit on the toilet, and then once he did, he sat up on the bed for over an hour, refusing to lie down to sleep. And that meant I couldn't go to sleep either. He can't be trusted to be awake in the house by himself. He could pee or poop anywhere, move things around, or try to brush his teeth with a razor blade instead of a toothbrush. That razor blade incident scared the hell out of me. He put toothpaste on it and was putting it up to his mouth when I stopped him.

I told him three weeks ago that if he peed on the floor one more time, we'd have to move him to assisted living. And now we really do have to seriously explore this option. I know that assisted living will make Richard give up, but I think he has already anyway. He has no fight in him. And I don't have much left either.

11 December 2014

Another difficult night with Richard. He fought me for fifteen minutes about sitting on the toilet. He insisted that it was OK to pee in the closet and was very angry that I was angry. I really don't know how much I have left in me.

The other day I was helping Richard get dressed, and I suggested he wear jeans. They were in one of the drawers in the closet. He told me they were wet. I opened the drawer, which was about the same height as the toilet, and damn if he hadn't peed in the jeans drawer and then closed it again. In some ways it was funny—but not really funny at all. I was impressed he remembered. He stated this as fact, not as anything other than that.

Earlier this week, we started work with a certified brain injury specialist, Katherine Lackey. Her work should help with making connections across different parts of Richard's brain and improve his neuroplasticity. As with everything else, I pray it will help.

Sometimes I wish it would all just end. Assisted living seems to be my only real option. Assisted suicide looks impossible. When Richard first started talking about suicide, I thought we could move back to Washington, as it's a death with dignity state, but that's not a possibility. The person needs to be of sound mind and have a terminal illness and less than six months to live. But he doesn't have any of those things. Richard asked me several times to help him kill himself. I told him I was truly sorry, but I couldn't help him with that, as I would go to jail. The Washington legal route was not for us. He understood but was disappointed. There will be no happy ending to this story.

I Want My Husband Back, but He Can't Make It

26 December 2014

*My best friend and love for twenty-three years
    has Parkinson's disease and dementia
It seems long ago when we were happy and
    healthy
Full of joy and adventure
Blessed with a life of travel and good fortune
Many were envious
The perfect couple
Smart, good-looking, and so in love
Now I'm your caregiver
Worried about bowel movements and falling
    and gluten-free diets
And making appointments, hoping without a
    scene or backing out at the last minute
We tried everything to get you back to health
Or at least to slow the vicious decline
Friends and strangers tell me how strong I am
But I don't feel strong
I feel exhausted and sad and angry and alone
Richard moves to memory care next week
High-end lodge in a desertlike place
With a view of the mountain we love
Maybe he'll thrive there or simply wait to die*

Tears of despair, prayers for a miracle, and armies of professionals don't change the harsh reality
I've lost the man I married somewhere along the way, slowly and day by day. At first, I didn't notice
Sometimes he's still here. A tender kiss, a quiet thank-you and I love you
I want my husband back, but he can't make it

They say that there is a reason for everything, but it's probably just a bunch of crap to make those who suffer feel better.

Moving Out

January 2015

I discovered there are people who specialize in finding care facilities for your loved ones—like a real estate person for those with special needs. This is a fantastic notion and a tremendous help. Margaret Roberts came to our home to interview us and determine our needs. She made all the appointments and drove us to each of them. Oh my God, she was a lifesaver. I am entering a new world with so much to learn.

Richard moved to a beautiful and brand-new memory care facility in Oro Valley on December 31, 2014. We liked it because it didn't feel like assisted living. It had more of a resort feel, with great views of the Catalina Mountains and lots of activities. It snowed the day Richard moved in. Here's the view from his room. December 31, 2014, was the first time I had a full night's sleep in months.

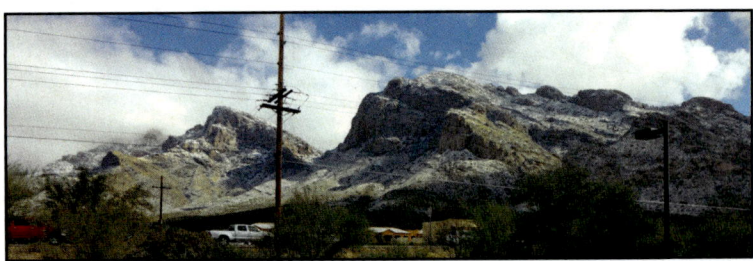

Here's the email I sent on Christmas Eve, 2014.

Dear family and friends:

Despite oceans of tears and hours of prayers—many of them from complete strangers—and our using nearly every intervention available on earth, Richard's health continues to decline. The dementia remains our biggest opponent, and it's winning. The Parkinson's continues to progress rapidly as well. It's impossible for him to focus or communicate coherently or manage his personal care.

So with great sorrow, I tell you that Richard will soon move to a memory care home. The one he chose is a brand new, high end lodge-in-the-desert-like place with great views of Pusch Ridge in the Catalina Mountains.

For the most part, I stopped working for the last year, but I need to get back to it soon. I have daytime caregivers, and that helps a lot, but it's the intense level of personal care and especially the challenges of the night that are causing me to make this decision.

We've been grateful for our army of medical professionals and our great friends and family. I'm not sure what 2015 will look like, but hopefully Richard will thrive in his new setting. And for myself, I know that consulting is far easier than caregiving.

This isn't a very nice Merry Christmas Eve message, but I wanted you all to know at the same time. We so appreciate all your love, support, and prayers.

Much love to you all.

Ava (Sue)

He was kicked out three weeks later. He became agitated, and they didn't give him his clonazepam fast enough. He hurt his neighbor's wife accidently, and it escalated from there. They called the police, and Richard was restrained and sent to the emergency room. It was awful. When I met him at the hospital, he was screaming. It was devastating and broke my heart. He calmed down when he saw me and finally got the clonazepam. But his new facility wouldn't take him back.

He was home with me for ten long days, including the time that his mother and brother were visiting for her ninety-third birthday. It was hell. We couldn't do much because Richard was still traumatized. And it rained a lot—good for the desert but not for out-of-town guests.

As you can imagine, Margaret was not happy about our traumatic adventure. She was a wonderful advocate for us and jumped to action to find a new place. Thanks again, Margaret.

March 2015

On February 5, 2015, Richard moved to Via Elegante, a much smaller and more homelike place. It has only ten rooms and ten residents, with two caregivers during the day and one at night. But he needs a private caregiver from 9:00 a.m. to 7:00 p.m. to watch over him and keep him active and out of trouble. This costs thousands of dollars every month. Plus, there is his work with Katherine, who helps tremendously, and weekly lymphatic massages with Susan. And just this Wednesday, we added acupuncture with Maryanne. She is very zen and great, but that's another cost. I think about Richard all the time and pray for him to be calm and happy. Sometimes he is happy. But not very much. Me either.

We've been blessed with a lot of guests. My brother and sister and families. My mom and dad. Friends Jeanne, Sue and Pat, Chuck and Lynn. Many people love us. I'm grateful for that.

Charming Richard is making friends with some of his fellow residents. Some aren't too amused when he walks into their room and takes a rest on their bed, but in general he is well liked. Another resident, John, has taken special interest in Richard. One night, after his private caregiver left for the night, Richard decided it was time for a stroll. According to John, he was minding his own business watching TV in his room, about to change channels, when he felt his wheelchair start to move. It was Richard, who had decided that

John should go for a stroll too. They were spotted in action by the night caregiver as he made his rounds. John loved telling me the story the next day. He clearly enjoyed the adventure.

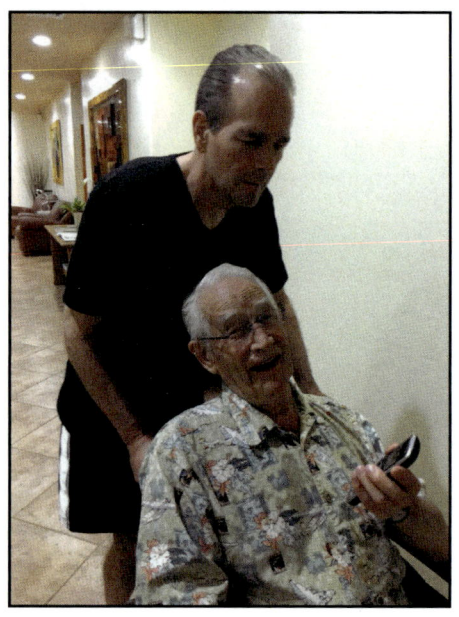

19 May 2015

As I read all this, I'm shocked at all that has happened in the last years. It's so fast and so terrible. I wouldn't wish this on the worst person on earth.

I went to our friend Ric's wedding in Palm Springs last weekend. It was so great to see him, and it's such a happy time for him. But I had mixed emotions. It was the first time I had traveled to Palm Springs on my own and the first time I stayed at the Parker without Richard. He loved that hotel. I'm not used to being on my own so much. But it's been coming on for a long time. I better get used to it.

26 May 2015

It was five years ago today that Richard was diagnosed with Parkinson's. I would have never guessed what would be in store for us. When we heard the news, I thought, *So what? His hand will shake a little bit.* But Richard's dementia was something we never expected, and we were not warned about at all. It wasn't even mentioned. The first year wasn't too bad. We tried so many things, and they have definitely helped. But it's been a very rough ride.

Twelve Ways My Dear Husband's Dementia Has Taught Me to Be a Better Consultant

21 June 2015

> Article for the Michael J. Fox Foundation and my business blog at Avasbutler.com

I am an organizational development consultant specializing in transformational change. I'm also the wife of my dear Richard. We've been happily married for almost twenty-four years and are deeply in love. But our relationship is a nontraditional one because Richard has Parkinson's disease and Lewy body dementia. In January, he moved into a memory care facility. He's sixty-three, and I'm fifty-seven.

Richard was diagnosed with Parkinson's in 2010, but we're sure he had the disease long before the diagnosis. We were somewhat prepared to take on the physical challenges of Parkinson's but utterly ill-equipped to deal with the accompanying dementia. Richard's decline has been rapid and relentless despite our full-scale attempts to do everything possible to stop or even reverse his disease.

Our situation has been devastating, but it has made me an even better consultant and person.

Here are the top twelve things I've learned, or relearned, so far.

1) Watch for early signs of problems.
   - It's easy to dismiss or ignore information that you don't want to hear.
   - Rely on those around you to provide insights. Ask for feedback.
   - Listen to what others have to say, regardless of whether you see it yourself.
2) Learn as much as you can.
   - Educate yourself, even on topics that you don't want to learn about and may have trouble understanding.
   - Pay attention to the details and don't be afraid to ask for clarification when people are speaking in a language foreign to you.
   - Get ready to be an advocate.
3) Get the system in the room.
   - Insist on a cross-functional, multidisciplinary approach and create opportunities for people with diverse views to hear and learn from each other. This is essential in order to determine the best solution or approach.
4) Plan ahead.
   - Last-minute changes to your priorities due to

unforeseen circumstances are inevitable. Expect and accept them with grace.
- Never wait until the last minute to get prepared. It will add to your stress and the stress of those around you.

5) Plan for all scenarios.
- Most people plan ahead based on predicting a few different scenarios. But few plan for or discuss the most devastating possibilities, and therefore they might find themselves in emotionally and financially difficult situations that could have been avoided or diminished.

6) Be flexible.
- Plan to manage current and known future priorities, but you must also adapt to your changing environment.

7) Pre-position others beforehand.
- No one likes surprises. Advance communication, sometimes several times, before an event occurs helps individuals prepare.
- Always avoid personal surprises in public places. Never let a person be embarrassed or humiliated due to your actions or inactions. Honor the self-esteem of others.

8) Show compassion.
- Be understanding and know the limitations of others and yourself.
- Listen carefully to maximize your understanding of others' situations and perspectives.

- Be present in the moment.
9) Focus on the positive.
    - Negative feedback, especially when it's focused on capabilities that another doesn't have, is counterproductive at best.
    - Think about what you and others can do, as opposed only thinking about what you or others can't do.
    - Look for creative solutions to maneuver around obstacles.
    - Celebrate even the smallest wins.
10) Take care of yourself.
    - As they say on the airplanes, "Put your own oxygen mask on before helping others."
    - Accept the help of others. Don't be afraid to ask for help and do so proactively.
    - Find joy in your work.
    - Remember to breathe.
11) Help others.
    - Share what you have learned and mentor those in earlier stages of their journey than you are.
    - Give freely of your time and know that your goodwill will be returned.
12) Be grateful.
    - Appreciate what others do. Say thank you a lot.
    - Treat every day as if it were your last.
    - Make a difference every day. Have a positive impact on those around you.

I'm still learning, whether I want to or not. I'll continue to work to be the best consultant I can be and the best wife I can be and to become a better person because of it. Transformational change indeed.

Letter from Mike

19 August 2015

Dear Richard:

It was really great to see you last week. I enjoyed seeing your place, meeting Joey and the others, playing basketball with you, and having lunch at Saffron. (I should have ordered what you did!)

My flight home was uneventful, but it gave me a lot of time think about our friendship. Brother, it has been a long, fun ride with you and will continue to be. I think back to the days when you went to Evergreen Jr. Hi. and I went to South Jr. You were a stud BBaller, and I thought I was. Then we both ended up at Cascade, and as sophomores we started to connect. You were on the baseball team (although you really didn't like Coach Krause), as was I. But it was beyond sports that I saw this great friend in the making. We started hanging out, going to each other's houses, chatting, and being guys.

I loved being at the Ping house and really liked Vernon and Marilyn and put up with Jim because he was a senior and I had to. (Since then, Jim and I have formed a great friendship, thanks to you!) I admired your peaceful nature and musical talent. We were in choir and swing ensemble together, but you were a real musician; I just sang. But basketball, man, you were the man!

I remember the first time I smoked pot was with you and we went to the end of the Paine Field runway, a little loaded, and watched as one of the first 747s took off as we lay on our backs at the end of the runway. Security was a little looser back in those days. I remember a lot of summers hanging out, talking about girls and sports.

By the time we were seniors in high school, we were very close but had to say goodbye like a lot of other friends as we went our ways to colleges. You to Central for hoops and me to Pacific for baseball. Our hopes and dreams for big professional paydays as athletes were short-lived but we ended up at Central together.

Then we began this cycle of not seeing each other for periods of time but always reconnecting. At first, I thought I was losing my friend every time you moved, but then I realized that we were living our lives but would always reconnect. When you met Ava, became engaged, and then married, Cathy and I were excited for you and wanted to get to know this babe you so dearly loved. And guess what? We found out quickly why you felt about her the way you did. You were great intellectual matches and complemented each other in many ways. So we saw you here; we saw you there. Seattle, San Diego, Vancouver, Tucson, London, etc. And you know what? That is what friendship is about. It took me a while to realize that when you and Ava moved, I wasn't losing friends; I was just getting prepared to hear about new adventures that fascinated me and made the bond even stronger. We never abandoned each other; we just took sabbaticals.

When we had our 40th high school reunion, I was so glad that you and Ava made the trip to Everett for the event. People were so glad to see you and meet Ava (I actually think more of the latter). But I knew there was something not quite right. I knew that you were sick. But I also knew that you were blessed with two things—you were a fighter, and you had Ava. You were going to do your best to fight this nasty invasion of your health. And you have been a fighter. You have put up with a lot of treatment, pain, frustration, confusion, progress, then not.

Believe me, brother, I think of you all the time. I think of what I can do to be there for you. I think of our friendship; I think how tough you have been. I think of what you want to say but can't. I think of what you want to do but can't. But guess what? Just like when you were a sophomore in high school and most folks didn't believe that no way in hell this skinny kid could make the varsity basketball team, much less start, much less be a star in the league, you did it because you are gritty. Still are. And I love that about you.

So, my buddy, I enjoyed my stay in Tucson last week. It was great to see you and Ava. She loves you dearly—so do I.

Mike

Coming Home

December 2015

I live in a condo on the second floor, and the woman below me died of Parkinson's back in July. Mary lived there with live-in caregivers. I could tell she was an elegant woman with style. But it's hard to be elegant and with style when you have advanced Parkinson's. You drool and can't sit up straight.

She couldn't walk and was always in a wheelchair. Once, when Richard was still living at home, we were outside and said hello, as we often did. I told her that Richard had Parkinson's too. She looked at him with sadness in her eyes, as if to say she was sorry that his life would end up like hers. She couldn't talk at all, but she didn't have to. I knew what she was thinking. I think Richard did too.

One day in October, it occurred to me that if I bought that condo for Richard, we could feel more like a family again. I could not *not* do it. I thought it would be cost-neutral, but that was self deception so I didn't get scared away from the idea. I found Mary's son and bought the condo. It was already close to move-in ready, but I had it renovated to open up the kitchen so caregivers could see Richard in the living room when they were in the kitchen. It has the exact same floor plan as our condo upstairs, but with beautiful hardwood floors and handicap-accessible bathrooms and showers. We painted it with warm and calming colors.

You can't see the mountains from the ground floor, but it's got great light and views of our courtyard—good for spying on the neighbors. I had reflective window film put on our windows, so they couldn't spy back.

Richard moved in on December 15, 2015. His assisted-living place threw him a party, and he was really moved. When you are in assisted living, all the other residents and their families and caregivers become your family. You're all in it together to make what is sucky less sucky. Sometimes it's even fun. Not that often, but it's possible. For sure you care about everyone there.

Richard loves his new space. I told him he was in charge of the ground floor, and I was in charge of the second floor. We have two twelve-hour caregiver shifts—7:00 a.m.–7:00 p.m., and 7:00 p.m.–7:00 a.m. Someone is awake with him 24/7.

And I love it too. It is so much easier to spend time with Richard. I can stop by between meetings and several times a day instead of having to plan a block of time sometime during the day. Visiting at night when he was in assisted living was a waste of time—Richard usually went to sleep by seven. And his cognition and energy are usually worse as the day goes on.

We put Richard's bedroom in the quietest room, in the middle of the hallway, directly across from the best handicap bathroom. It is cozier, so Richard feels safer than he would have in the master bedroom at the end of the hall. That room has sliding glass doors to the back patio, and any sound from the nearby driveway would have left him in fear of intruders. Putting his music room and guest room at the end of the long hall will make the house easier for Richard to navigate. Ha!

I moved a lot more of our art (we have a lot of art) and some furniture downstairs, more than he was able to have in assisted living. It felt like home—or as close to home as we were going to get. Richard liked having more of our stuff around. These photographs were taken by our dear friend and photographer Daniel Moret when we on a holiday together in Paris many years ago. They are "very important photographs," according to Richard, and I agree. He looks at them often.

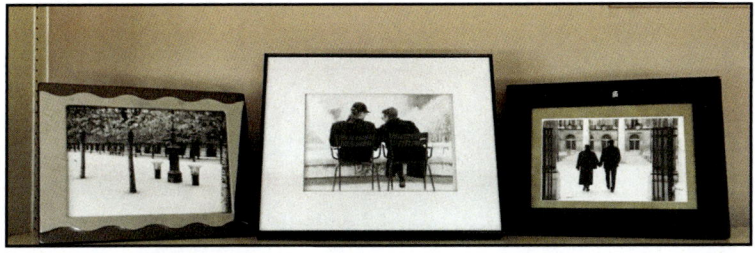

The house always smells good. A diffuser with lavender in the bedroom to help Richard relax and sleep. The diffuser in the living room usually has peppermint to help keep us focused and alert. And there's sage nearby to help with anxiety and shoo out the bad guys. Open the door, out you go. "Only the divine are welcome; all nondivine must leave now and forever." Cate taught us to say that. She's a healer and often clears our house of negative energy that Richard feels acutely and me not at all. I swear dementia gives you powers that the rest of us don't have. "Sleep with the angels, Richard." I say that to you every night.

The caregivers feed us great food. This is awesome. Of course, I have to buy the food, but for a person who hates to cook, this is a wonderful gift. The caregivers just text me to say food is on the table, and I'll come down. I love that.

I spend as much time as I can downstairs. Richard comes upstairs too, but that involves stairs, so it has to be a good day for that to happen. Stairs require a lot of concentration and coordination. Richard has jobs to do, like taking out the garbage every day. It's important to have a purpose and responsibilities, no matter who you are. Of course, we go with him when he is outside. Better to have two people with him, one caregiver and me. That way, if he gets spooked and starts to run or fight against us, we have a better chance of managing him. Bad boys can show up anywhere and at any time.

The Roly-Poly Visitor

28 April 2016

Several friends and even doctors have been saying that Richard should have a companion dog. My response has always been the same: hell no. I hate dogs. OK, *hate* is a strong word. How about *despise*? Let's just say I don't like dogs. In general, Richard doesn't either. He was a real estate appraiser before he sold his business and had many run-ins with dogs. Once Rottweilers that were supposed to be chained up ran after him, and he had to jump a high fence to escape. One bit at his leg and ripped his jeans. In short, dogs are not for us.

But they have worked on me—our sinister, dog-loving friends. They brought over their pets for visits. Suddenly, we were having homeless dogs coming over for dog dates with their foster humans. Then one day, a diligent woman from the Arizona Poodle Rescue brought a dog from Phoenix. She had brought over other dogs for dog dates before and was very tuned in to Richard's special needs. Much to my chagrin, we had become her project.

The dog she brought this time seemed nice enough—abandoned, in need of a new home, and with a horrible traditional poodle cut. He is male, thought to be about eight years old. I was under the impression it was to be a short visit, but the poodle lady said the dog should stay with us overnight because if we didn't like him, he'd have to go back to Phoenix the next day. Damn. I have been duped. Tricked by a dog lover. She brought dog treats and food and a collar and leash. A f'ing starter kit.

But this dog knew immediately why he was here. He doesn't seem to know anything about being a dog, but he does know he is here for Richard.

I had only told Richard that a dog was coming for a visit, not that it would be staying. He didn't like surprises. I would usually prepare him for days before something big happened. And this definitely counted as something big. So I asked Richard if the dog could stay. I called him the visitor. "Would it be OK if the visitor stays overnight? He doesn't really have anywhere else to go." Richard said OK.

Kathy, our weekend caregiver, calls him the roly-poly visitor, because the dog is quite plump. He had been overfed by his foster family. Richard seems to like him well enough. As Richard was getting ready for bed, I asked him if we should give our roly-poly visitor a name. Richard immediately said, in an unusually strong voice, "Tacoma." And Tacoma it is. Richard had lived in Tacoma, Washington, for many years, and we all think it is a fine name.

Tacoma is a major pain in the ass. He doesn't know that he is supposed to pee and poop outside. No idea that this is important. Because he had been abandoned, we don't know his background, but we were told he was abandoned twice in life, when he was young and again just recently. The poodle rescue people knew that based on his chip. Tacoma is terrified of being abandoned again. He won't even walk away from the house unless Richard is with us. I have to pick him up and carry him. Very frustrating. I've hired a trainer, and Al is teaching me and Tacoma a lot. The dog is for Richard, but I have to do all the work. I don't hate Tacoma, but I don't really like him either. But he is here for Richard, and their relationship is growing. Tacoma wants to be everywhere that Richard is—in the bathroom, by the table, watching TV. He often sits on Richard's lap. This is an awesome trick to get Richard to sit still for longer. They are good buddies.

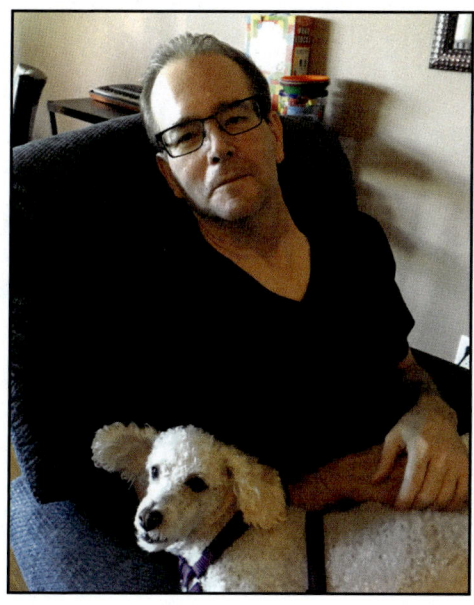

Tacoma charms everyone. He is quite cute, especially after a morning at the spa. "The perfect accessory," my neighbor Linda says.

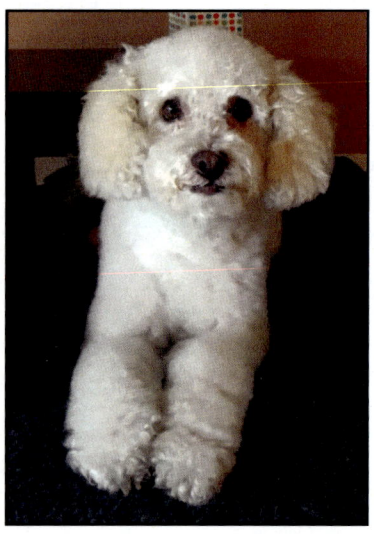

When Richard gets sick, Tacoma gets sick too, as if he is trying to take the burden away. It is super annoying, but his intentions are good. It didn't take long to figure out that Tacoma is an angel disguised as a dog. He is pretty bad at being a dog, but excellent at being an angel.

Basketball

Richard was a fine basketball player. He started with the varsity team when he was a freshman in high school, and it was his passion. His friend George put it this way: "Richard did things that no one else did. Hit the open man, dribble through *any* defense, and hand out jockstraps after the drive."

When he blew out his knee in college, he was devastated, and he never truly recovered. We shot hoops together a lot over the years, and he was a passionate Washington Husky basketball fan.

Parkinson's puts serious constraints on one's body. Arms don't swing like they should; people stoop over, take tiny steps, and get frozen in place. Richard has all those challenges. Big time. But put a basketball in his hands, and he turns into a different person. He becomes much more agile, with better posture and balance. Muscle memory is an amazing concept. We play ball almost every day. As Richard's diseases progresses, we can't use the basketball hoop as much, but it makes a nice lamp.

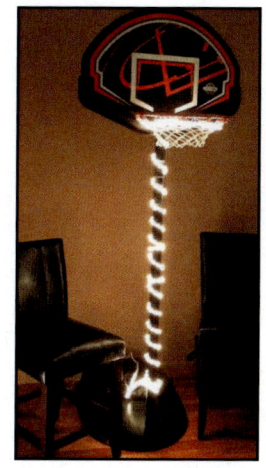

When friends and family come over, we always play basketball, passing and bouncing the ball to each other. It puts Richard on an even playing field with the rest of us. He can't hold his own in a conversation. That is impossible. But with basketball he is as good as or better than the rest of us. His self-esteem rises because this is something he is still good at. It is fun, a good social activity, and a good workout. More than once my arms end up burning, but there is no way I will stop if he isn't ready.

Sticker Charts

To keep track of Richard's most important activities and accomplishments of the day, we use a weekly sticker chart. Dr. Pam, Richard's psychic healer, had this idea, and we have expanded upon it. It's a great way for me to keep tabs on how each day and night are going, and it also helps caregivers coming onto their shift.

Richard and I review the week's sticker charts together, looking for categories that went well and categories for improvement. It gives Richard a sense of accomplishment. He pays attention. Sometimes we look for trends over the last weeks.

Every category is important. Water intake is huge. Constipation is always an issue for people with Parkinson's. So are having good posture, using a voice loud enough to be heard, going outside for physical exercise, doing puzzles for brain exercise, and taking naps.

Richard was an excellent musician, and he has a piano and two guitars. We encourage him to play every day.

Caregiver Joey is a musician too, and on good days they have great jam sessions together. There are extra stickers for that. Richard named their band Land Work One. We liked that name. Here is their band photo.

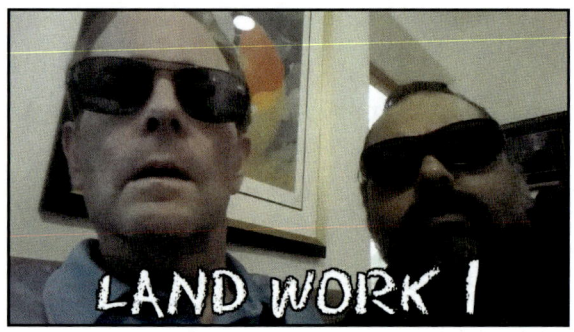

At first, we used cupcake stickers for poops. It entertained the caregivers and me. After a successful poop, the caregivers would yell out "Cupcake!" with the exuberance of a sports announcer exclaiming, "Goooooaaaaal!" at a World Cup match. There were lots of cupcake jokes, and Joey's were the best—or worst, depending on your interpretation. To this day, I don't eat cupcakes.

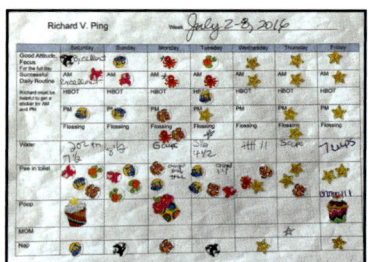 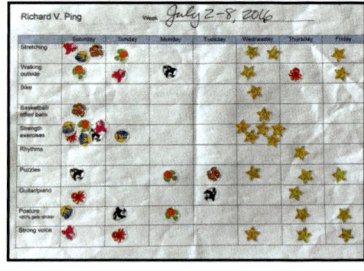

Then we moved to dinosaur stickers. Large dinosaurs, large poops. This was even more informative and entertaining.

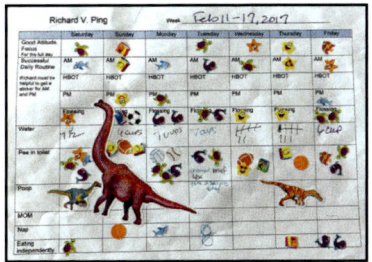 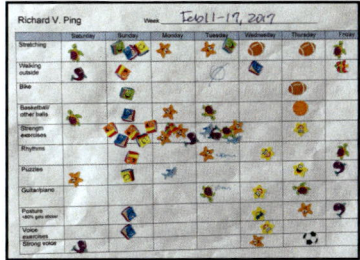

After Richard passed, caregiver Abbra's daughter made me this present with the extra stickers I gave her. As you can imagine, I love it! I call it Richard's Poop Pot.

There are days when I wish I was giving myself stickers too, with different categories. Maybe I'll do that.

Lies!

I walk downstairs and walk through the kitchen door. I immediately sense that Richard and the caregiver are at odds.

Elsa states what happened in frustrated terms. Richard has not been cooperating and is therefore in trouble. From across the room and in a loud voice rarely heard, Richard yells, "Lies! Lies!"

Elsa and I both burst out laughing, at both the rebuttal and the strong voice. In most cases, Richard apologizes (after a serious conversation with me); the apology is accepted, along with compliments on his strong voice.

But my dear Riccardo has trouble staying on his best behavior. It won't be long until he is again defiant, either because he doesn't like being told what to do (never did, no matter how nicely) or is too unfocused to comply with instructions.

Richard is not good at being a cooperative patient. He hates the very idea of needing assistance. Sometimes he calls out, "Jim, Jim!?" when he feels he needs reinforcements.

We explain, "Unfortunately Jim is not even in the same state as us and therefore cannot come to your rescue. It is to your advantage to cooperate so we can finish faster, and furthermore Jim would agree with us."

This is not the news he wants to hear. He's been known to cuss at and fight against caregivers who are simply doing their job to help him sit on the toilet, get in the shower, get dressed, or whatever else they are trying to do on his behalf.

Luckily most of the time, he's still kind and charming and funny. Damn good thing, or we'd have no caregivers.

Dementia for Dessert

Sugar will kill my husband. Not directly, as with a gun, but as a malicious and seductive accomplice. Alzheimer's is called type 3 diabetes, after all. And sugar sure as hell isn't helping our situation.

Richard loves his sweets and has done so since he was a little kid. He would sometimes eat a whole box of sugary cereal in one sitting until the top of his mouth was sore. Or devour four packages of M&Ms at a time. This was not good.

Once when we were having dessert with friends in Italy, Richard asked for a bite of friend Ambra's profiterole. It was the last one the restaurant had. It was so delicious that it was as if he went into a trance. He ate the whole thing so fast that no one else got a single bite, including Ambra. He apologized about that for years.

After I read *Grain Brain*, by Dr. David Perlmutter, we moved to a gluten-free diet. That has not been hard, but keeping Richard away from sugar is another thing. He loves his ice cream and gets very crabby if I try to deny him. He'll eat a big bowl of ice cream, and within a few hours, his cognition is far worse than before. It is so predictable that it is annoying. As his dementia gets far worse, however, it isn't as noticeable.

So as Richard's Parkinson's and LBD has gotten to the point that he can't reliably swallow pills, we open up the capsules or crush the pills so that the ingredients are only powder. The powder goes over the first scoop of ice cream and then gets covered up by the second scoop. This is further hidden with lots of organic dark chocolate syrup. The perfect disguise.

"Swallow your pills please, Richard" has a 0 percent chance of success.

"Please eat your ice cream, Richard" has a 100 percent chance of success.

When life gives you lemons, make lemonade. Or something like that.

The Last Year

19 April 2016

Richard, today you were standing in the hallway, and you looked like my husband, the old you. That was really wild and beautiful to see, if only for a minute.

6 July 2016

Today is our twenty-fifth wedding anniversary. What a crazy ride. I haven't written in so long, and much has happened. I bought us a bottle of Veuve Clicquot, our favorite champagne, but Richard wasn't that interested. It wasn't one of his better days. The first time Richard bought me a bottle of champagne, it was Veuve Clicquot. And we've been drinking it ever since. We always bought a case at Thanksgiving, and it usually lasted us until New Year's. But if not, we'd just buy more. There was always something to celebrate. Drinking it now just makes me sad.

20 July 2016

Our anniversary was a very hard day for me. Yesterday was my birthday, and that was hard too. I had wanted to go on safari for my sixtieth birthday, combining it with our twenty-fifth anniversary for a big adventure. We went to Ireland for Richard's sixtieth birthday. Richard chose Ireland; I chose a safari. There will be no safari. Not now. Not together.

That aside, I certainly didn't expect to be in the situation we are in. Not in my wildest dreams. I don't regret it and know I am here for a purpose, but it's one that I could have done without. I was very happy the way I was.

Managing the house is a lot of f'ing effort. But it's becoming a fine-tuned machine.

Managing our finances is beyond tricky. Richard would shit if he realized the big nosedive we are in. He'd be livid. My consulting work has taken a big hit since I gave up my happy life as a road warrior. I only work locally now and not nearly enough to get ahead. I often tell people it's a good thing I love my husband as much as I do, or I'd be really pissed about the costs. But like I said, I could not *not* do this. And I'm scared to death.

I miss being with you alone, Richard. I miss sleeping in the same bed together. I miss our cuddles and affection. Sometimes we dance together, especially in the mornings after your shower, when the caregiver is making us breakfast. I love that. You still have some moves. And sometimes your kisses still take my breath away.

30 August 2016

So many couples live together in unhappiness for decades. But Richard and I are deeply in love and are being robbed of our time together. I hate the irony.

25 September 2016

My dear sensitive husband and his caregivers are not allowed to watch or listen to the news. Ever. It upsets him. If someone got shot, he's afraid we'll get shot. If there is a house on fire, he's concerned that our house could catch fire too.

But there are lots of sports to entertain us. March Madness is the best, of course. Formula One races. Horse races. When American Pharoah won the Triple Crown, I thought he and Kathy would blow a gasket (whatever a gasket is). Winter and summer Olympics. The World Cup. Track and field. Men and women, college and professional sports. There is always something to watch.

We watch either sports or nice TV, like the documentaries about adorable baby animals or movies with happy endings. That's all that is allowed. Last December, Kathy got Richard hooked on Christmas movies. I can't stand them, but they both got teary at the gushy, sentimental parts.

And there is lots and lots of music. Favorites include Joe Bonamassa, Frank Zappa, Pink Floyd, and Santana.

We start every day rockin' out. We have classical piano to settle us down. We have music for every occasion and situation.

Perhaps we should all live our lives this way. Forever the poet, Richard said just other day that we are "living in the days of thunder." Truer words were never spoken.

2 October 2016

My dear husband has Parkinson's disease and Lewy body dementia. It's taken over our lives. I fight a battle every day that I will not win. He won't win. We just make the most of what we have and try everything at our disposal to prolong his inevitable fate.

Some say I'm a fabulous wife. Some days I think I'm a fool. Richard's ending won't be fast, and it won't be pretty. It will be costly and emotionally draining. No drug will save him, and although there is hope for future generations inflicted with these diseases, it's too late for Richard. I can make it the best it can be, but it won't change the outcome. I know that, and everyone else knows it too. I'm doing the best to manage the change that nobody wants. And it sucks.

Sure, there are many things to be grateful for, and I am. But it sucks and has fundamentally changed my life in a way I didn't want and have a hard time being cheerful about.

But I have to keep going. I have to provide for our

family and for myself. I have a lot to manage, and I get up every day determined to make it work. There is no other choice, whether I like it or not.

I'm not alone in this challenge. There are millions of caregivers and soon-to-be grieving widows and widowers just like me, with every imaginable background and story.

Managing the Change That Nobody Wants

10 October 2016

Article for the Michael J. Fox Foundation and my business blog at Avasbutler.com

I'm an organizational development consultant who specializes in helping business leaders achieve transformational change; it's my life's calling.

But not all change is wanted. My dear husband, Richard, lives with Parkinson's disease and Lewy body dementia. It's costly, time consuming, and emotionally draining. No currently available drug will cure him, although there is hope for future generations.

There's an irony to unwanted change happening to the change expert. Though my background provides helpful skills and experience, I'm in uncharted waters. I learn every day. And I've got a long ways to go.

Here's some of what I've learned so far about dealing with a change you don't want but can't avoid.

Keep the beautiful moments in the forefront of your mind.

There are plenty of painful moments that threaten to take over your consciousness. I try to balance upsetting thoughts with those of the tender kiss that still takes my breath away, Richard placing his hand on top of mine, and his beautiful blue eyes when they still twinkle. Or the way that his face lights up when a caregiver's daughter sings a song she learned that day.

Be grateful for the big and small acts of kindness that others show you.

Be vulnerable enough to let people you know—or complete strangers—help in ways you would never ask for or even think of.

As they say on airplanes, "Put your own oxygen mask on before helping others."

You cannot help if you are burning yourself out. Take the time to go out with friends, take a walk, or do whatever makes you happy or gives you a break.

Be kind to yourself.

You will make silly mistakes due to stress and big mistakes because you didn't know any better at the time. Try not to beat yourself up.

Don't be afraid of medical terms or of not understanding the doctors.

It's their job to explain things to you. Ask questions and paraphrase back to ensure understanding. Ask again and again until you feel comfortable with your understanding of the information you need to manage your situation.

Know that others are facing challenges or grieving too.

And they might say or do things that aren't helpful. But they are trying to do what they think is best. In the event that someone's attitude or advice is not helping you at all, don't hesitate to ask for space.

Do your best to accept your new normal.

There is no point in expecting your life to be like it was before the disease or like those of your peers. Your life is different and special now. Do what you can to enjoy it.

For us, international travel was a big part of our lives. We can't do that anymore. But we can take a trip to our local mountains for an hour.

Help others like you find their way.

Take the time to connect and share with others. I've been able to help others who are at different places in their journey. In turn, they support me too.

Pray for the best and plan for the worst.

You want the best for your loved ones and yourself. Miracles do happen. But I also focus on sobering things like financial planning and preparations for if and when Richard needs a wheelchair.

There are millions of people managing unwanted change, with every imaginable background and story. I hope my advice can help others, and I look forward to hearing others' reactions and suggestions.

We Tried Everything

When traditional medicine let us down, we did not give up there. We tried everything. Everything has helped, but nothing has been a cure. That would have been a dream. Here's the list of the things we have tried:

- Acupuncture
- Cognitive therapy
- Counseling
- CBD and medical marijuana
- Fisher Wallace stimulator
- Gluten-free diet
- Hyperbaric Oxygen Therapy (HBOT)
- LSVT Big
- LSVT Loud
- Massage therapy, lymphatic massage
- Meyer's drips with glutathione
- Neurologists
- Neuro-pharmacologist
- Psychic healers
- Pharmaceuticals
- Physical therapists
- Stem cell replacement therapy
- Supplements

Once when Richard was at the office of his acupuncturist, Kym, he got up off the table when she was in another room and walked out on his own into the street. With the needles still in him. Luckily Kym saw him and rushed out to say, "Hey, Richard, where are you going?"

"Going home," he said.

"Why don't you come back inside and we'll wait for Ava," she said this in a normal voice. Then she calmly got his needles out and sat with him in the waiting area until I returned. They chuckled about it later. But to state the obvious, I was not allowed to drop him off and pick him up after that. On-site guard duty was required.

Nuplazid came out for Lewy body hallucinations in June 2016, and it has been a gift from the heavens. Richard still sees extra people, but they aren't nearly as scary. Pity it didn't come out years earlier. Life would have been a bit smoother.

Landing the Plane Safely

We have tried some wild stuff and working with Dr. Pam is high on the wild stuff Richter scale.

Dr. Pam is a psychic healer and a damn good one. Our main goal is for Richard to "land the plane safely" in this lifetime so that his anxieties, fears, and unresolved issues—and mine as well, for that matter—do not follow us to another lifetime. I want our next lives together to be on a higher level of peace and power. I'm not doing this again.

Dr. Pam works with Richard's spirit guides and connects with his higher self to help him address issues getting in the way of leading the best life possible. Her own spirit guides help too, as do other archangels and whoever else she summons.

One of the first times we met with her, Richard was looking over Dr. Pam's shoulder as he started his session. (I was allowed to sit in because Richard was rarely able to communicate clearly due to his condition.) Dr. Pam asked, "How many fairies do you see, Richard?"

"Four," he responded.

"I see four too, Richard," said Dr. Pam. I, of course, saw zero fairies, but just because I couldn't see them didn't mean that they were not there. I was the least evolved person in the room.

Dr. Pam has worked with Richard and with me for over two years. And it has helped a lot. Oh my God, has it helped a lot. And we will eventually land the plane safely.

Told you it has been wild.

The Cold That Killed My Husband

22 April 2017

On March 15, I had a reading with Dr. Pam. Richard had visited her virtually earlier that day and told her that he couldn't do it and that he wanted to go. His plan was to choke to death. He told her he thought I would be better off without him. That part isn't true, but that was his opinion.

For whatever reason, he couldn't make the leap to healthiness. God gave him the chance, and many angels and archangels were there to help, but he wasn't able to. I forgive him for that. I just pray that he is at peace. My goal was to land the plane safely in this life, so he could be at peace in the next one. That was my only goal.

I had a terrible cold and cough, as did half the population of Tucson. The cold that killed my husband.

Richard caught my cold on Friday, March 17, and in typical fashion it was dramatic. Thankfully none of the caregivers got sick. Just him. An omen. Michelle, his Friday night caregiver, said this one was different. She didn't like the sound of it. And she'd seen him sick many times before.

He continued to get worse and had a chest x-ray on Monday, March 20. I was so grateful that Dr. Bravo ordered the chest x-ray to be done at our condo. There would have been no way to get Richard out of the house. Sitting in offices was difficult even on the best days.

On Tuesday, the results came back showing a lower respiratory infection, and I knew it was the end. Just the day before, I had a feeling I should reread his living will. It had an amendment that told me exactly what we had to do. Richard had insisted we have our wills done back in 2008. I'm so grateful that he did.

In part, here is what the addendum said.

If and when I am no longer mentally competent and there is little or no likelihood that I will regain mental competence as determined by my physicians, I not only request but demand that in the event of infections, including pneumonia or other serious infections, I do not want parenteral antibiotics or oral antibiotics that in any way could be interpreted as life-saving...I wish to reemphasize that when I am no longer mentally competent, it is my wish to die in a normal course of events without benefit of medical intervention.

Pretty damn clear. No arguments about the path forward. Decision taken.

Richard was too sick to get out of bed. He was basically dead weight, and Elsa and I couldn't get him up by ourselves. He still weighed 160 pounds. On Tuesday, Joey came on his day off to help move him. Together we—mostly Joey—got him to the shower, where he had a gigantic poop. An *Argentinosaurus*. We cheered, once again grateful for poop. It seemed strange at the moment. But even if you're dying, you need to poop. All the caregivers were so wonderful. We were blessed with such a great team.

On Wednesday morning, Dr. Bravo came and was concerned about Richard's oxygen level, which was 75–80. She ordered Casa de la Luz hospice that day, and everything was set up that afternoon—hospital bed, oxygen tank, morphine, that horrible but wonderful sucker machine to get the phlegm out of his throat, pills, and so forth.

He got progressively worse, and on Thursday the hospice nurse told me that he probably wouldn't make it until Monday. I was grateful for the warning.

Our dear friends Mike and Cathy came on Thursday and left on Friday morning. Brother Jim and partner Sophia arrived on Friday afternoon, and family Steve, Sandy, and Anna came for the day on Saturday. It was wonderful that they were here to say goodbye. It was March, and we often have out-of-town guests that time of year. Another blessing. All were planned visits, but Jim and Sophia hadn't planned to come for three more weeks. I told them Richard won't be with us in three weeks. They dropped everything to get here the next day.

Richard completely stopped eating and drinking by Thursday. The hospice nurses said to let him take the lead. If he wanted to eat or drink, he would. Tacoma stayed on the bed with him, and that was a comfort to Richard—and probably for Tacoma too. Tacoma knew his job was to be there for Richard up to the very end.

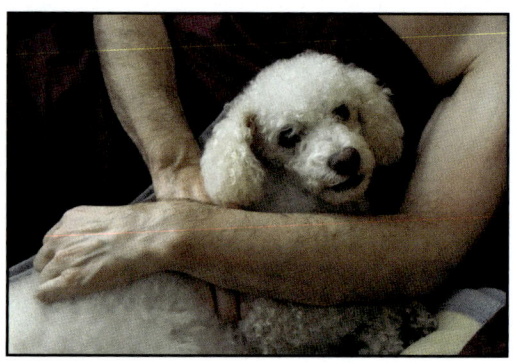

The hospice nurse came again on Sunday morning, March 26, at 9:00 a.m., and said that this would be the day. His oxygen level was down to 60. Hospice nurses are angels on earth. Richard's eyes hadn't opened for days, his breathing was terribly labored, and the experience was beyond surreal. "Today's the day," I said to Richard, holding his hand and gushing out tears.

On Sunday around 10:35 a.m., Richard opened his eyes and stared out, looking directly at and through me. I was so grateful to see his beautiful blue eyes again and to tell him how good our life together had been and how much I looked forward to our next life together. We were all there in his bedroom together—me, Kathy, Jim, Sophia, and Tacoma. All crying, of course. Then my dear Richard died at 10:37 a.m.

Once Richard passed away, his face looked so

peaceful, and he was back to his handsome self. I found great comfort in that. The hospice nurse and Kathy dressed him in his best Washington Husky clothes. I wanted to take a photo but thought it inappropriate. But I don't need a photo. I'll remember that moment forever.

The funeral guys, very nice young men, took Richard to the funeral home to be creamated, and then we were left alone. Poor Tacoma was forlorn, and we were all very sad. I prayed that Richard was at peace. I was sad but at peace knowing that this was what he wanted and that he no longer had to suffer.

Many have since told me that pneumonia is an old man's best friend. For us, that was true.

Richard wasn't old, but it was his best ticket out of town.

Tacoma's Too-Big Promotion

April and May 2018

After Richard died, the question was what to do with Tacoma. He couldn't stay with me, as I'm gone too much.

Andy, the owner of Via Elegante, Richard's last assisted living place, offered to take Tacoma as the house dog for his facility in Sierra Vista. It would be a big promotion, as there was not only the one house with ten residents, but three houses all with long hallways in between. But unfortunately, there were no doggie doors. There were managers to help make sure he got his food and medicine, but since he roamed between the three buildings and gave no indication that he had to go out, he had frequent accidents inside.

After two months, he got fired—mainly for peeing next to people with catheters and barking at spirits. The staff call them permanent residents. I thought his antics were amusing, but the staff did not.

Then he came home with me again. I told him the universe said we weren't done with each other yet. He stayed with me for a few weeks, and I did learn to love him in the end.

Now he's found his perfect home, with colleague and friend, Nancy and her golden retriever, Gracie.

Gracie taught Tacoma to act more like a dog, and for the most part, he has no accidents. He has even learned to play with toys, which he had no concept of before. He's retired from caregiving, but he's still an angel disguised as a dog.

It's Different to Grieve the Death of a Loved One When They Have Been Sick for a Long Time

27 June 2017

For OptionB.org

It's different to grieve the death of a loved one when they have been sick for a long time. It isn't as shocking, and it includes a sense of relief that the suffering is over.

But I'm not sure that it's easier, though. The grieving starts years before death. And that's tough for sure.

It was June 2010 when my dear husband, Richard, was diagnosed with Parkinson's disease; a few years later, he was diagnosed with Lewy body dementia. I knew what to expect with Parkinson's, but I'd never heard of Lewy body dementia and didn't anticipate the impact that its hallucinations and delusions would bring. I was new to this game and didn't know what the future would hold.

As early as 2008, Richard started being more anxious. As one example, he suddenly developed a fear of flying. Despite first-class tickets and flawless flights, he would spend the ten hours of an international flight checking his watch roughly every three minutes—every one to three minutes for ten hours. That's really hard to do.

Paranoia and anxiety were never far away after that. Hallucinations and delusions dominated our world shortly thereafter. From 2015 on Richard needed professional care and was in assisted living for a year, before I bought the condo below me for Richard and to allow for 24/7 caregiver support.

Dementia and Parkinson's are horrible diseases. I don't wish them on anyone. But as with any other challenge in life, they do provide an opportunity to learn and grow, whether you want to or not.

It's been over three months now since Richard's death, and I'm bridging to my next chapter of life. I had been a caregiver and "extraordinary" wife for so long, always taking care of every detail. And now that's over. A bit of a shock, really.

Now Richard's spirit takes care of me, and I feel him every day. He's much happier to be rid of his uncooperative body and the limitations his diseases brought.

We had such a great life together. It was filled with beauty, adventure, lots of fun, and a deep and lasting love. Richard taught me to be a better person, although I wasn't really that interested in being better. He still considers me a work in progress and continues to teach me kindness, patience, tolerance, and unconditional love on a daily basis. He keeps me smiling and reminds me not to take myself or life too seriously. I am so deeply grateful.

N 48°08′, W 123°00′

23 July 2017—Richard's sixty-sixth birthday

Around four o'clock on Sunday, we headed out to sea from the John Wayne Marina in Sequim for about thirty minutes, as Jim, Sophia, and I drank champagne and told stories about Richard.

Richard's mom didn't come, as it would have been too hard for her to get on and off the boat.

When we were a few miles out, the captain cut the engine, and we all said silent prayers and teary goodbyes.

Then I dropped Richard's urn into the water, which caused a gigantic splash, getting me completely wet. We all burst out laughing.

Jim said Richard did the best cannonballs of anyone as a kid. He clearly wanted a big send-off.

Then we put five roses in the water for Richard— white ones from me, Sophia, Jim, and Mom/Marilyn, and a red one from Dad/Vernon, who had his ashes placed in the same area thirty-five years ago.

Vern led the way and guided them all out to sea with the tide. All the white roses stayed in a line, with the red one first in front, then to the side, and later guiding them from the rear once getting back in the line.

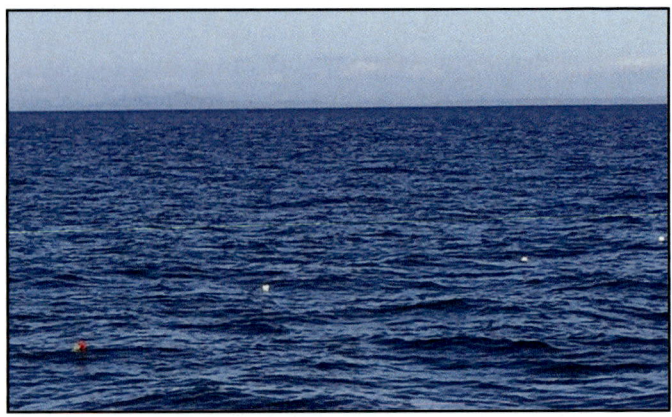

The captain later said he'd never seen anything like it. We watched the roses float out for some time, said goodbye, and headed back to the marina.

It was a beautiful day.

August 2017 and January 2018

We had no funerals but many celebrations. The biggest one at Mike and Cathy's house the evening before Richard's birthday. That one especially meant a lot to Richard and me.

I'm spreading smaller portions of Richard's ashes at his favorite places.

Friends Les, Sue, Debbie, and Roger joined me to spread ashes on the fourteenth green of his favorite golf course, Vistoso in Oro Valley. Richard used to play there four days a week for years and loved the course.

Some ashes are at the cliffs of Point Loma, California, where we loved to watch the ocean and the pelicans flying by. For some unknown reason Richard loved pelicans.

More ashes are spread at the top of the Peak Chair at Whistler. It's a scary chair scaling the side of a cliff with an excellent view at the top. Cathy didn't want to take the chair to go with me, but she did it out of love. It does seem perilous.

We loved Whistler and had a time-share there for over twenty years. We skied a lot of places in the world, and Whistler is by far our favorite. When the 2010 Olympics were there, they placed an inukshuk at the top the mountain. Here's Richard's view from behind the snowy inukshuk.

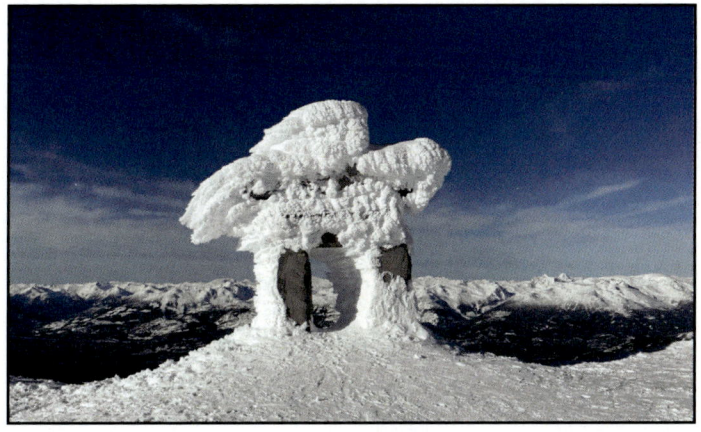

More ashes will go to Richard's favorite city, London; his favorite country, Italy; and the place of his heritage, Scotland. I just haven't gotten there yet.

Life without Richard

26 June 2017

It's been three months today since Richard passed, and I feel sad today. So many people love Richard, and we're all grieving.

But there is peace in knowing that he no longer has to live with the indignities his body and brain caused him. He was a very dignified person, with awareness of his situation, and he hated it.

I'm so grateful for all the kindness, love, and support we received over the years. It's been incredible and not to be taken for granted.

Death does not end a relationship, and our romance continues, yet in another form. The great book *Option B* talks about posttraumatic growth. I'm going for that. It's not easy, though.

I really miss Richard, and I expect I always will.

I also miss being fed by our caregivers every day. Another loss, but one that's far easier to adjust to.

26 August 2017

Now it has been five months, and I feel sad and lonely today. Sometimes it's just too quiet.

Abbra had her baby on June 21, and his name

is Noah Makhi—a strong name. She asked me to be Noah's godmother, and I was thrilled to accept. Abbra was Richard's primary night caregiver. She worked Sunday–Tuesday, from 7:00 p.m. to 7:00 a.m. Richard liked her. Her then-five-year-old daughter was having troubles staying with other family members when Abbra worked, so I invited her to bring Nevaeh with her. Nevaeh was very shy at first, but she and Richard quickly became friends. They would toss a ball back and forth to each other, and Richard adored her. He said she was the prettiest girl in the world.

Here's Nevaeh's crumpled drawing of them playing ball.

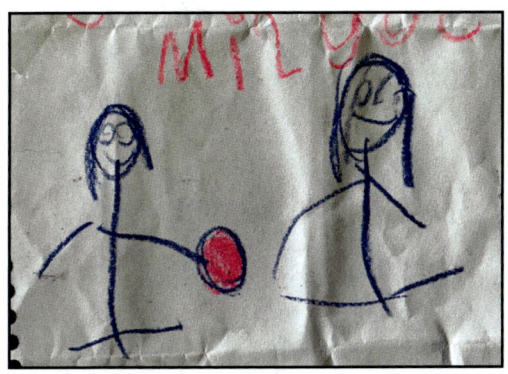

Abbra and Nevaeh were with Richard during his last night on earth.

Richard was the first to tell Abbra that she was pregnant. As she stood next to him while he sat on his bed, he leaned over to put his ear against Abbra's belly and listened. She was surprised by his action. She found out three days later that she was pregnant.

14 September 2017

I find it very difficult to be alone. Having Noah around helps so much, but he's not with me often. Here's a photo of the happy little guy.

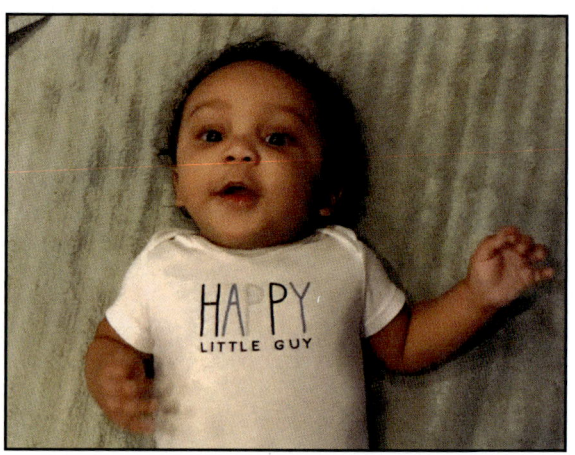

I ask myself why this is happening and what I am to learn. It appears that I must learn to rely on myself and know that I am enough. So I am saying this mantra today: I am whole by myself.

I must focus on the future and not the past. I am spending too much time thinking about emptiness and aloneness and loss. This must change today.

The universe seems to be telling me to write a book, and I'm trying not to listen. It keeps coming up in thoughts and conversations. I'm not sure about a book, but I want to keep writing for sure. I have many articles completed, and I plan to put them together. Perhaps

I could create a blog and a website, including letters from friends and photos. The path will reveal itself.

26 November 2017

It's time for me to blossom. But blossom into what?

Today is the eight-month anniversary of Richard's passing. I still feel empty and can't imagine how life can be full and complete without him with me in this world. But I must release myself from old pain and open myself to light. The light of Richard, the light of us, the light of the universe. I am ready. At least I hope so. This is getting old.

December 2017

Christmas is kicking my ass. I was having a good day yesterday, and then I realized that this would be the first time in twenty-six years that Richard won't sign holiday cards with me. That made me cry. Even last year he signed our cards, albeit creatively. I'm surprisingly distraught about this.

I keep looking at my front door, hoping that my dear handsome Richard will be standing there ringing the bell, saying "Congratulations you passed the test with an A- and now I'm back good as new." Like in one of those damn Hallmark movies.

Friends Allison and Rich adopted me for Christmas day, and I'm grateful for that. My work projects have finished for this year, and I expect and pray to gear up again in January. It's good for me to keep busy. But if

I'm too busy, I don't take the time to focus on my feelings. I hate that.

28 December 2017

Well, for the most part, the holiday sucked, but I've been feeling a bit better since Christmas Eve. It got easier to write holiday cards as it went on. I would have skipped the whole thing, but I have so many people to thank for their love and support. I'm not very productive at all, but I guess that's OK. I'm doing a lot of healing, it seems. So that's a good use of time.

I do pray to be able to work a lot in 2018. I really need and want to. I enjoy my work, and I'm good at it. And I really need and want to start building up my net worth again.

7 March 2018

I committed to myself and to Richard yesterday that I would create a website and blog of some sort that share our stories with the purpose of helping others.

2 May 2018

On September 14, 2017, I wrote in my journal that I was told to write a book. Today, when I was hiking Tumamoc, I finally decided that I would do it. I envisioned a *New York Times* best seller for nonfiction. I already promised Richard on the anniversary of his death that I would do something. But I've been dawdling.

I basically argued with Dr. Pam when she predicted that a change would come to my career. I said I wanted to make money. Well, I'm not. So here I am again, being pushed—my guides would say directed—by the universe to get out of my comfort zone again.

7 May 2018

I'm starting to write this book, *Parkinson's: A Love Story with Dementia for Dessert*. It's going to be a lot of work, and it will make me cry. I'll be reliving my past pains. Over seven years of them—more if we start with anxiety and depression from 2009 and even before. But I know I have to do it. Good books don't come without effort.

I know the universe is telling me to do this, even though I'd really like to just be a regular consultant again. But nope, that's not an option. So here I go, growing again when I don't want to. I'll treat it like a job. Damn universe.

I'm Afraid of a Day

7 March 2018

I'm afraid of a day: March 26. That's the day that Richard passed, at 10:37 a.m. It will be a year. I'm afraid just thinking about that day. I'm afraid about how I will feel and what I will do. It's not rational. I know what the pain and loss are like already. I know what it's like to be alone and sad. But I don't know what I will do that day. I must accept these feelings. I cannot block them. It won't make it a bit better. It's just a damn day, but I dread thinking about it.

It's just a day on the calendar, but it's the last day I held my dear Richard in my arms and saw his beautiful blue eyes and kissed him. It's the day he left behind all the pain and despair and anger of his disease. The day he went to live with the angels. It's the day that the wonderful hospice nurse and Kathy gave him a bath and put on his favorite Washington Huskies clothes and the day that the young men from mortuary came to take him away from us. It's the day that Tacoma knew he lost his job. It's the day that all the caregivers lost their jobs.

It's the day that years of pain and fear were over. I was relieved for Richard and also for me. I didn't know how much longer I could hold on. The stress was intense. But so is our love. And that's the part I remember the most now: our love.

Of course, the pain wasn't over. Not then, not now.

I'm afraid of a day: March 26.

Holding My Breath Doesn't Help

2 May 2018

Holding my breath doesn't help. It doesn't work at all really
I know because I tried for years
Tensing up muscles in anticipation of the hurt
Squinting my eyes hoping not to see harsh realities so clearly
Fear of fear. Afraid of pain and the energy required to face it and to let it go
I have two good reasons: Parkinson's and Lewy body dementia
My dear husband Richard's illnesses and death took so much out of us all
Fear of not knowing how to manage, knowing it would never be enough
Knowing there would be no happy ending
Fear of not being able to provide. Not being able to stop his pain. Or mine
Fear of living without him. Fear of being alone
It's hard work to hold one's breath for years
A failed attempt at suppression. Delay of inevitable truths
But suppression of the bad also means suppression of the good
The joy and beauty of life can get sidelined

Not noticing when birds sing and children laugh
Gratitude diminished or forgotten
I'm slowly letting go of the fear and pain
And feeling lighter, with eyes open wider
Breathing more freely and deeply
Someday it will be my norm

What Does It Feel Like to Be Dead?

12 May 2018

Ciao, Riccardo, what does it feel like to be dead?

Staci Wells, another fabulous psychic I've worked with since you passed, says you are at peace. I can feel that. When you left us, you were ready. Your struggle was becoming so hard. She says you have a sense of overwhelming relief at the personal freedom and joy you have been experiencing since you woke up on the other side.

But it took some time to rest and recover from the built-up toxicity from your life here on earth. Now you share love from your heart every day. You give something to someone every day. You are bringing light to others. I wish we all did that.

Staci says you're still playing the piano on the other side. It was arpeggios when we last spoke. You asked to play Staci's piano while we were talking. That made her laugh. It must be a good piano. You were a bit of a snob about things like that.

She says you are whole on the other side and dancing. You are complete. That's beautiful, Richard. I'm so proud of you.

I feel you sleep with me at night, our souls entwined.

I feel you flying beside me when I'm hiking. I note how much more you enjoy hikes now that you can fly. When you were a human, hiking hurt your knee.

And I feel you flying beside me when I'm skiing. No more worries about your knee here either. I sense you're doing fancy, show-off flips. Cool that you do that, Richard, you recovering smart-aleck daredevil.

I talk to you a lot and ask you to give me angel advice. So far, I mostly like what you tell me. Sometimes I resist, but the universe is on your side.

I can hear you most clearly when you are angry with me. *Calm down*, you said when I was getting huffy with my parents. *Slow down*, you say when I drive too fast. *Are you f'ing kidding me?* when I park the car poorly (again). *Get the damn kid to basketball practice*. OK, I'm doing it.

As the Grateful Dead say:

Sometimes the light's all shinin' on me,
Other times I can barely see.
Lately it occurs to me what a long, strange trip
   it's been.

Lately it's occurred to me what a long strange trip it's been. No shit. It's been a wild ride for sure, and one that I will always hold dear.

OK, Deadheads, I know you're singing "Truckin'" right now, aren't you?

Living with Grief: Truth Versus Fiction

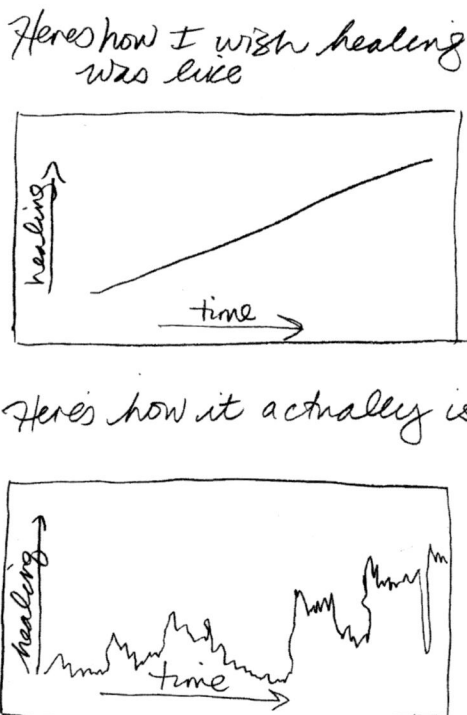

Rats, that sucks. And I'm told it never ends. Maybe one day, I'll get used to it.

My Very Own Cardinal

17 May 2018

Here's a piece of beautiful folklore shared by my dear friend Andrea:

> A cardinal is a representative of a loved one who has passed
> When you see one, it means they are visiting you
> They usually show up when you most need them or miss them
> They also make an appearance during times of celebration as well as despair to let you know they will always be with you
> Look for them, they'll appear

And look, here's Richard on the tree outside my balcony—high in the sky, with the jacaranda tree blooming for the first time since we moved here.

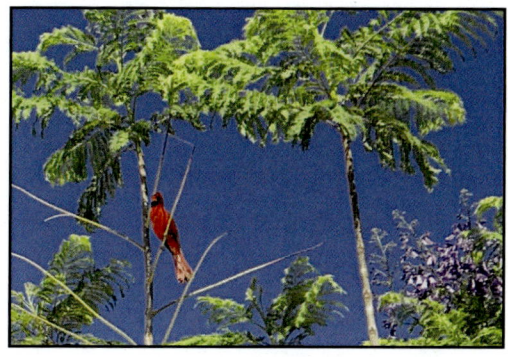

Neighbors say it's blooming for the first time ever. He's been here flying around for a few weeks, and I love it. He makes me smile, pause to be in the moment, and feel deeply grateful every time I see him. He was here last summer too but never for this long.

The female cardinal is close by too. She stays even a little closer. Richard is coming to me as the yin and the yang, female and male energies. They both sing so beautifully all day. I think it's a good sign that I am healing. Time for celebration, damn it.

Happy Birthday, Dear Richard

23 July 2018

Today you are sixty-seven, my dear Richard. You stayed with me on the earth until you were sixty-five, and we met when you were thirty-nine. That's twenty-eight years so far. I opened a bottle of Veuve Clicquot and poured two glasses. Cheers to you, my best friend and the love of my life.

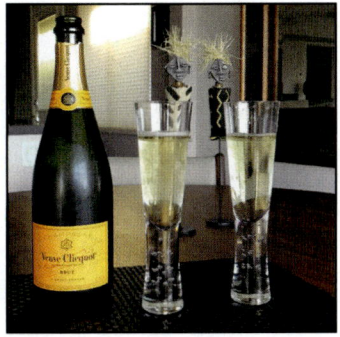

Every day I miss you being on the earth with me. But I find great comfort knowing that your spirit is still with me every day and that you have found peace and contentment in heaven. Now you can radiate pure love without the shackles of your diseases. I know you will be there to welcome me with open arms when it's my time. I look forward to that day.

In my mind and in the minds of all who know us, you will always be the handsome man you were before you got sick. My favorite 2011 photo of you is on our tall bedroom dresser. I lean on the dresser with my head on my arms and talk with you every day. I will get old and even more wrinkly than I was in our

Halloween picture, and you will always look like this. It's not really very fair. I'm the vain one, not you.

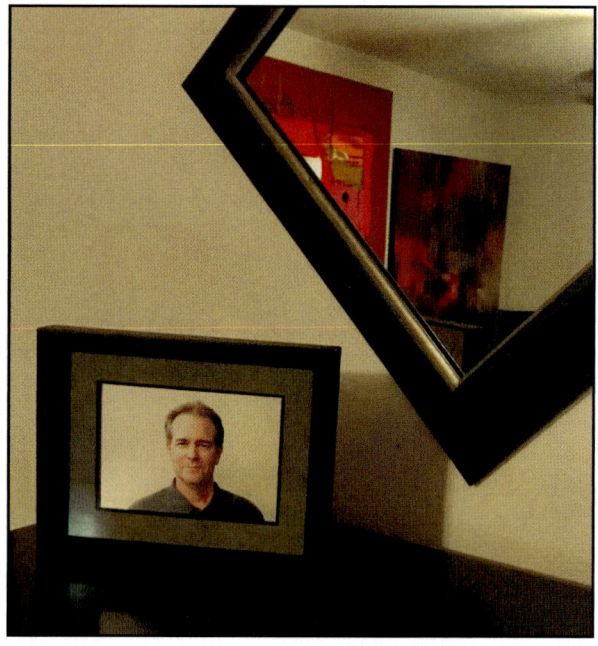

PHOTO OF RICHARD BY PURPLE NICKLE

I'm so grateful that you are in my life. I wish it would have been an easier path, but I know that it couldn't be any other way. I'm still on my journey of healing and know that it will take this entire life. It hasn't been easy, but I am grateful nonetheless. What else can I do but choose posttraumatic growth? If I don't evolve now, I'll be left to deal with it in another life. We've got better things to do the next time around. "Land the plane safely," I said. Now it's time for me to fly the plane again. Knowing how well you are doing, I've got some catching up to do.

But it's not easy. July is kicking my ass as we could

have predicted it would. We have our twenty-seventh wedding anniversary on July 6, my sixty-first birthday on July 19 (I still want that damn safari), and now your birthday today. This was always our month of celebration and adventures.

If there was not an adventure, then there was another piece of art. I love our art and the fond memories it brings me. You loved our art too, and your great taste kept me from buying crap I would later regret and that you would cuss for eternity. A few months ago, I did buy a little seven-dollar mask from Mexico at my favorite rest stop between Tucson and San Diego—the one with hundreds of trinkets and big metal horses and dinosaurs. I always insisted we stop there. I heard you swearing in disapproval, but I couldn't resist the prank. "Ha ha, can't stop me," I said out loud, making the lady next to me stare.

"God damn it," you replied. The lady didn't hear that part.

I'm grateful for the beautiful lightning storms of our monsoons and for Noah and his family. He's thirteen months old already. I visited him at daycare today, and he ran to me with open arms and a big smile. That made me happy.

I'm grateful for our wonderful friends and family and for our new great-nephew, Ozwald Michael, who is already one month old. I'm going to strive for favorite great-aunt status, but the competition is fierce. You would be the favorite great-uncle, no contest, and probably still could be. Start working on your angel magic tricks.

I'm sending our book to the publisher this week. It's been painful, but I'm glad I'm doing it. Thanks for all your help, my word wizard spouse.

I'm grateful every day I see the cardinals that now reside here. You delight the whole neighborhood. Stick around, please.

Oh my God, what a long strange trip it's been and will continue to be. In our wedding vows, I said, "Grow old with me, Richard; the best is yet to come." This was true, just not in the way we first imagined. Not the way we imagined at all. But love stories come in many forms, and we were soulmates—and still are, of course.

For resources and more information on
Parkinson's and Lewy body dementia, please visit
www.DementiaforDessert.com

Made in the USA
Middletown, DE
20 December 2022